Yoga's Path
to Weight Loss

A Mind Body Spirit Guide
to Loving Yourself Lean

Kathleen Kastner, M.S., Exercise Physiologist

Transformational Wellness Publishing

© 2015

Published by Transformational Wellness Publishing

Book design by Lorna Moy-Masaki

For my sweet Dad, Bob Kastner,
who is free of his body and always with me in Spirit.
I love you for eternity.

"Yoga means union; the path of Yoga is the science of uniting the soul with God."
—Paramahansa Yogananda

Contents

Section 3: Food

Chapter 1
Introduction

And I said to my body, softly, "I want to be your friend." It took a long breath and replied, "I have been waiting my whole life for this."—Nayyirah Waheed

Do you want to lose weight, have glowing skin, and love yourself more? If the answer is yes, this book is for you! Losing weight is one of the things in life over which you have total control. Every day, three times a day—breakfast, lunch and dinner—you get to make the choice of what you put in your body, and how much. No one is holding a doughnut to your mouth forcing you to eat; you decide. You also get to choose whether you exercise each day or not. Most importantly, *you* hold the power over the beliefs you have about your body and yourself. All of these choices begin in the mind. This is why it is important to have mindfulness tools to help you make conscious healthy choices.

I have been working in the health field for over two decades as an exercise physiologist, personal trainer, and yoga teacher, observing thousands of people in their quest for improved health and weight loss. During the sixteen years I was a yoga studio owner, I saw more people lose weight with yoga than I did when I was a personal trainer. I wrote two articles about yoga and weight loss, entitled, "How Yoga Can Help You Lose Weight" and "Liberation from the Gym: The Magic of Ashtanga Yoga." The response was positive: male and female readers both wrote me with similar stories. Many

ॐ 1 ॐ

had quit the gym, like I had, and were losing weight and feeling better from their yoga practice. Their support is the inspiration behind this book. I realized there was a large population who needed an emotional and spiritual approach to weight loss to lose weight permanently, not just diet and exercise tips.

My weight loss formula is based on what I experienced in my own body and the bodies of my students and clients through the years. My program is for people who want to improve their health, lose weight, and deepen their spiritual connection while having fun along the way. Yes, weight loss can be fun and enlightening when you learn and apply new, life-transforming practices.

My approach isn't about drinking protein shakes, taking supplements, counting calories, or eliminating carbohydrates. It entails eating a wide variety of plant-based foods, including desserts, along with simple disciplines that can easily be adapted into your daily routine.

Because you are more than just a body, these daily disciplines use the mind, body, and spirit to make this a holistic approach to weight loss. In traditional weight loss programs, the number one focus is always on the body—eat this and do these exercises—but the body isn't the problem. The mind needs discipline, and the soul needs to be healed.

Addictions begin in the mind. The body is just following what the mind tells it to do. As the saying goes, "As above, so below." Let me give you a few examples:

- Do your arteries want animal fat?
- Do your lungs want cigarette smoke?
- Does your liver want alcohol?

- Do your adrenals want caffeine?

If the body had a voice, like in an animated movie, I believe the answers to all of these questions would be, "No." Unfortunately, the body is being drowned out by the voice of the mind, which in a state of weakness will often times say, "Yes."

The good news is, deep inside, you have the consciousness and self-discipline to reverse unhealthy habits and replace them with positive lifestyle changes that will help you manage your weight for life.

My program will help connect you to this higher state of consciousness and the God of your knowing through yoga, prayer, meditation, journaling, affirmations, and walking in nature. All of these practices will deepen your union with God. I use the word "God" because that is what resonates with me. Feel free to replace it with whatever word resonates with your belief system: Universe, The Divine, Mother Nature, Spirit. It's all good.

To participate in this program you will need:

- Yoga Mat. I recommend a Manduka Pro-lite Mat. They are sturdy, nonslip, and have a lifetime guarantee: www.manduka.com. Cheap yoga mats have a lot of plastic in them and can turn into a slip and slide, making it hard to practice.
- Yoga clothes or exercise attire.
- A pair of walking shoes.
- If you have physical limitations that won't allow you to do yoga, try chair yoga.

ॐ 3 ॐ

- If you aren't physically able to walk outside or on a treadmill, I suggest riding a recumbent bicycle or participating in water exercise classes.

- The plant-based cookbook, *Oh She Glows*, by Angela Liddon, available at www.ohsheglows.com.

- A cushion for meditation. This can be one from your couch or bed. It doesn't need to be an "official" meditation cushion, unless you want to buy a special one or make your own.

- Optional: *Insight Timer* application to track meditation practices and the *Lose It* application to track calories and exercise.

- Journal for recording thoughts, feelings and affirmations.

- The motivation to cook for yourself. Remember, if you can read, you can cook.

- An open mind and a willingness to change!

THE BODY

ॐ 5 ॐ

Chapter 2
Your Body Is a Temple for Your Soul

The body is God's house.
—Pedro, Ace Car Rental driver

After returning from a week-long vacation in San Diego, I was headed to the airport in an Ace rental van. God orchestrated Pedro, a sweet Hispanic man in his 60s, to be my driver. The second I saw him, I could sense his goodness and the light in him. He was immediately kind and extremely patient with me. I notice these things about people who work with the public daily. Some people don't need yoga, because they embody yoga without trying.

On our drive to the airport, Pedro told me he used to live in San Diego but now lives in Tijuana, because he can get the same sized apartment there for $1,000 less a month. He was saving his money so he could move his family back to San Diego and buy a house. He worked two jobs, the first with Ace Car Rental, from 7 a.m. to 2 p.m. Then he worked at the car wash down the street from 3 p.m. to 11 p.m. After his long work day, he made the drive back to Tijuana so he could fall asleep and do it all AGAIN the next morning, while still wearing a sweet smile on his face. I asked him how his body could sustain a 15-hour workday. He replied, "I don't drink, smoke, or do drugs. The body is God's house."

Pedro's words sum up my book in one sentence: *The body is God's house.* I believe God individually created and designed each of our bodies as a gift to us, to house our souls and to enjoy the human experience. He also gave us free will to treat our bodies how we choose: with respect or disrespect. This is where self-love becomes a critical point in weight loss and how you treat the temple of your soul.

For years, I mistreated my body, and I learned a lot from that experience. Growing up, I over-exercised, especially with running, to compensate for my feelings of not being "good enough." I was adopted, and this was the story I created in my mind. At the time, I didn't realize I was abusing exercise, because I was too young to be conscious of my habitual pattern. Now, looking back, it is textbook to me. Someone later in life brilliantly asked me, "What were you running from?" Myself, of course.

Some people would pay money to have an exercise addiction, but trust me, it can be just as debilitating mentally and physically as not exercising at all. It's like having a tyrant in your mind, telling you to work out harder and faster, even when you don't have the energy or are injured. You've probably witnessed an exercise addiction in a friend or family member and the damage it can do, not only to their bodies but to their lives and relationships as well.

Starting in high school, I would run six miles a day, every day, whether it was a blazing hot Kansas summer afternoon or a freezing winter evening. It didn't matter, because my mind was wired so tightly there was no room for any other option. If I didn't run, my mind would tell me I was "less than," a loser. So running I went, no matter what my body said, even through throbbing knee pain.

Some days I would run to our local YMCA, do an aerobics class (this was the 1980s), go to the weight room for another hour, and then run home. Along with this unhealthy habit came addictions to sugar, tanning beds, picking my skin, and Diet Coke. My entire life was WAY out of balance, with underlying anxiety.

When it came to food, I was either over-eating—like my five bowls of cereal after my morning run—or under-eating—like my interesting lunch combo which consisted of a school cafeteria bread roll and a box of Hot Tamales from the vending machine. This routine carried over into my college years, where I managed to control my weight through exercise even with the addition of beer and pizza. My weight did fluctuate a bit at the end of my college years, but not much, because my mind wouldn't allow for it.

After I finished graduate school, I moved from Kansas to San Diego. I was born and raised in Kansas, so this was a big leap of faith for a small-town girl, especially because I showed up to California jobless. Rarely did anyone in my immediate circle of friends ever leave the security of the Midwest, but my soul was determined to fly the nest.

Thank goodness, I landed a job at a hospital wellness center...but the only catch was I had to open at 5 a.m., Monday through Friday. My 4 a.m. alarm was a rude awakening from my former late-night college years. Because I was grateful to even have a job, I took it joyfully. However, soon it started to wreak havoc on my health, due to exhaustion and my poor food and drink choices.

Things were slow on my early morning shift, so I looked forward to the morning coffee cart with its delicious scones and large mocha coffee drinks. I'm sure this combination made up about 700 calories, most of which were sugar. This would have been fine if it were a holiday or weekend treat, but not for a daily ritual. I continued to exercise, but it wasn't enough to compensate for the thousands of calories I was unconsciously consuming at work and at night when I went out drinking with my friends. I learned real fast that beverages are not calorie-free.

Looking back, I realize I was depressed by my transition to a new state and was emotionally eating and drinking alcohol to cope. I was also trying to keep a long-distance relationship alive, which was dying a slow death.

Within six months, I had gained 20 pounds, more than I had gained in six years of college. The saddest part was, I never saw it coming until I saw pictures of my full face. I had left college at 118 pounds, and was now up to 138 pounds, lickity split! I was probably the only person ever to move to San Diego, the land of the fit, who gained weight.

Happily, I met a tri-athlete at my job, and he helped me get back on track. I stopped drinking alcohol, exercised with him daily, and we ate healthy vegetarian meals together. I quickly lost the first 10 of the 20 pounds I had gained. Soon thereafter, the Universe blessed me with the gift of meeting Dr. Deepak Chopra at my 5 a.m. job. I became his personal trainer and his staff introduced me to yoga. Little did I know at the time that yoga would be a life changer for me on EVERY level. I went into my first class thinking I was just going to stretch a little and ended up tearing up in the final resting pose. My mind and body were still, and my heart was feeling on a deep level. It was as if God and my soul were saying, "FINALLY, she is still. Let the healing begin."

Chapter 3
Quit the Gym and Step on a Yoga Mat

If you heal the soul, the body will automatically be healed.
    —Paramahansa Yogananda

When I started yoga, I had no idea what it was about. I wasn't skeptical, just Kansas naïve. I knew it was a form of ancient exercise, but that was about it. I would later learn that yoga means "union" in Sanskrit, union between you and God. My first yoga teacher even told me her greatest goal in life was to know God better. Boy did I have a lot to learn.

During my first class, the postures were challenging for my insanely tight fitness body. I was immediately trembling and sweating in the most basic triangle pose. Because I had lifted weights half my life, I was saddened by the fact that I couldn't do a single yoga push-up to save my life. Humbling to say the least. I had created imbalances in my body from my fitness routine—strong here, weak there—and they were coming to the surface.

Even though I wasn't "good" at my first yoga class, I left feeling like a million bucks and couldn't wait to go back for more. The practice had moved emotions and energies that had been stuck in my body for years, even since childhood. I knew I had experienced a profound shift, and I wanted to explore where it could take me. As medical intuitive Caroline Myss says, "Your biology is a biography of your life." Our life's experiences and emotions are recorded in our cellular memory. I visualize the body as a glass of water with sediment resting at the bottom. This sediment represents the emotions and experiences we've tried fiercely to forget, ignore, or escape. While they might have settled to bottom, they are still buried in our bodies. They can't fully be forgotten.

When we start breathing, moving, and connecting in yoga, these memories often come flooding to the surface to be healed. This is one of the major reasons yoga is so effective for weight loss—it helps people get in touch with the root of their issues. A student recently told me that in his first Down Dog pose, he had a flash of having both of his legs broken in a car accident as a child. His yoga practice helped him to process the trauma and gave him a sense of closure with the accident. This is a powerful testimonial of how yoga can help people heal on a deep level.

Releasing emotions and energies that have been trapped in your body for years can help you lose weight, especially if the beliefs behind them are causing you to overeat. Yoga is like physical therapy and psychotherapy, rolled into one. It brings the darkness to the light to be healed, allowing you to experience freedom from the past and live fully in the present. It helps you shed layers of your life and in turn, shed layers of excess weight. I tell people, "Wouldn't you rather heal these issues now instead of twenty years from now?" It takes courage to step on a yoga mat, so be prepared for a life-transforming experience.

If you enjoy your current exercise routine and it is producing the results you desire in your body—and not causing injury—then keep doing it. Add three days of yoga into your program. If you are bored with your exercise routine or don't have one, yoga is a way for you to lose weight, stay fit, and maintain bone density that doesn't include pounding on the pavement, high kicking, or stressing your joints with metal plates. If someone had told me in my jogging/compulsive cardio machine years that one day I would chuck it all to become a full-time yoga practitioner, I would have never believed it. Yet it was THE best decision I ever made for my health and life.

In 1999, when I opened my first yoga studio, I decided to do a 30-day pilot study with myself, doing just Ashtanga yoga seven days a week. Before that point, when I was still a personal trainer, I had been practicing yoga four days a week. This was in addition to cardio and weights, which were a big part of my life and job. Therefore, I was afraid to give them up. However, they were hindering my yoga practice by making me tighter and decreasing my range of motion. My yoga practice was becoming more enjoyable and important to me, and I wanted to progress.

The guys I trained with at the time thought I was nuts for giving up the gym, because weight lifting was their religion. They asked me questions like, "Shouldn't you supplement your triceps with curls?" and "Aren't you afraid you're going to gain weight?" I had no idea what would happen, but I did know I was bored out of my mind doing cardio and weights. Plus, I had self-induced a thick, muscular build that was not my natural body type.

In the late 1990s, when Spinning made its debut in the U.S., I would spin like mad and then wonder why my jeans wouldn't fit over my quads. I joke now that if I even look at a Spin bike, my legs blow up. In addition, all the intense cardio was making me eat the house down, because I was so dang hungry all the time. Once again, a lack of balance in my life. If you love Spinning, this doesn't mean you have to stop. Do what you love. Add in some yoga to lengthen out your muscles and bring a little peace to your life.

By the end of my 30-day yoga pilot study, my flexibility had improved, and I was feeling lighter in my body. My weight-lifting bulk had begun to dissipate, and my natural lean shape was resurfacing. No more quad wars. Most importantly, I was happier and eating less. I had zero desire to go back to the gym and have never since returned. Liberation from the gym is a beautiful thing, if you are bored with it. Again, if you love it or you're new to it, keep enjoying it.

In the years to follow, I lost 10 more pounds, quit smoking, quit drinking alcohol and caffeine, adopted a vegan diet, met my biological parents, and even met my husband in an Ashtanga yoga class when I least expected it. This is the magic of Ashtanga yoga. My whole life had a positive upheaval, an excavation of sorts. I could finally release unhealthy habits and see the truth of my soul, without hiding behind my physical body and compulsive behaviors.

One of my former aerobics friends later said to me, "*You haven't changed, you just changed subjects,*" meaning I was still an exercise addict, but now I was doing yoga instead. But I knew better. There had been a profound shift in consciousness that was carrying over into every area of my life. I was beyond grateful for this transformation.

When I was a personal trainer, I would also teach yoga classes at night. I noticed my yoga students were losing weight, but not my training clients. I began to realize why this was happening...and here's what I discovered.

Yoga changes your consciousness, your awareness, the way you think. Your thoughts become elevated due to the yogic breathing and stillness. With each deep breath, you are breathing in higher consciousness, which deepens your connection to your soul and to Spirit. Therefore, your decision-making processes begin to change in favor of honoring your body and life. An increase in self-esteem is inevitable. Yoga also makes you happy. When you're happy, you take better care of yourself.

Breathing is Spirit Moving Through You

As my Ashtanga teacher Tim Miller says, "Every time you breathe, you are doing a dance with Spirit." The breathing is what makes yoga a spiritual practice. Otherwise it would just be physical exercise. The breath is the bridge or link between the body, mind, and spirit. Basically, God is in the breath. This helps you connect the dots to all parts of your being, leaving you feeling more whole and complete and less fragmented. It makes sense that the breath also has the power to infuse and transform other areas of your life.

Yogic breathing is practiced with the lips sealed. You draw the air and energy up through the back of the throat, making a whispery "Haaaah" sound like the ocean, quieting the mind. This is called *Ujjayi*, or Victorious, breathing ("*jai*" means victory in Sanskrit). I like to interpret it as victory over the mind chatter and negative self-talk. It is different from nostril breathing, so think of it as nose and throat breathing, with sound. This audible sound gives the mind something to focus on during the practice. It is also a powerful tool to use in any situation that causes you stress and anxiety. Take a break from your life for a moment and inhale and exhale five slow, deep breaths while slightly constricting the back of the throat. Hear the whispery "Haaaah" sound, like you're fogging up a mirror, but with your lips sealed. This sound will help quiet your thoughts and calm your nervous system, which in turn can also help you control your emotions, cravings, and potentially ward off a binge.

Breathing consciously with the lips sealed causes the air to go up through the nose, where it directly links to the mind. This quiets the mind chatter and aligns the mind with Divine Mind, like in meditation. It then goes on to link your mind to your body and your body to your spirit. It's one big cycle of life force *(prana)* moving through you: breath, mind, body, spirit…repeat.

Every time you inhale with awareness, you are drawing in higher states of consciousness, helping to cultivate your Higher Self into being more prevalent in your life. Your Higher Self is the part of you that wants the best for you on every level and wants to put an end to self-destructive behavior. It reminds you that you are divine, perfect, whole, and complete just as you are in this moment. You are good enough. This is yoga's greatest gift: Divine love. Yoga helps you to love and accept yourself as God loves and accepts you, unconditionally. This is the main reason I want you to practice yoga daily, to infuse your mind and life with Divine love and self-love.

When you exhale with awareness, you are being liberated from tension, limiting thought patterns, and unhealthy habits that are no longer serving your highest good, such as addictions.

So the metaphor for yogic breathing can be summed up as follows: Inhale, drawing in new life force, healthy habits, improved self-esteem, and a deeper connection to Spirit. Exhale, releasing excess weight, fear-based thinking, negative self talk, and addictions. There is a saying in yoga: "Your bad habits will lose you." I have experienced this personally and have witnessed it in several of my students as well. More Divine love equals more self-love, which leads to more healthy choices in all areas of your life. Your inner world begins to reflect your outer world, so what isn't aligned with your truth tends to go by the wayside, especially when it comes to unhealthy addictions.

Here is an example: One of my students had a major chain-smoking addiction when she began yoga. After an intense class and a deep relaxation, she drove her usual 30 minutes home. By the time she got home, she realized that she had forgotten to light up, the way she always had in the past. "I made my entire drive home without my usual smoke. I just forgot," she said. The silence of her deep meditation had penetrated her consciousness and she no longer felt the need to smoke. Because she felt fulfilled from within, she didn't need her usual nicotine fix.

I also knew an 81-year-old doctor who wasn't able to exercise anymore due to physical limitations. He had read an article about the benefits of deep breathing for weight loss and had followed the suggested guidelines. He sat daily, doing deep breathing for fifteen minutes, inhaling through the nose and exhaling through the mouth. Over the course of two years, he went from 250 pounds to 204 pounds. He lost 46 pounds just by breathing 15 minutes a day, without exercise. He also reduced his meat intake to just one or two times a week, because he said his appetite had decreased greatly due to his breathing practice. He said, "I just wasn't very hungry anymore."

I suspect the prana—life force—in the breath, was fulfilling his appetite, like in the story of Giri Bala told by Paramahansa Yogananda in *Autobiography of a Yogi*. When Yogananda met Giri Bala, she was 68 and had not eaten or taken fluids for over 56 years. Chastised as a young girl for her hearty appetite, she prayed to God for help. God provided her with breathing and meditation techniques which allowed her to sustain her life force for many years without food and drink. Now, I don't suggest you stop eating or drinking, by any means. I just want you to be aware of the powerful effect deep breathing can have on your mind and body.

When I did conventional exercise, I never had the deep shifts in consciousness I have experienced in yoga. When I was focused on physical fitness, there was no dancing with Spirit, just unconscious panting with my mouth open. I was more in a state of hyperventilation than inspiration. It still pains me to see people running with their mouths open, huffing and puffing, a distressed look on their face. It doesn't look healthy, comfortable, or enjoyable. I want to let them know there is another way to exercise that can be peaceful and productive.

Yoga also brought me a sense of inner peace and self-love that I never found in the gym or on the pavement. I wasn't running from myself anymore; I was going inward and getting to know myself on the deepest level...and, surprisingly, I liked the person I found. It also taught me how to eat to live, not live to eat. It taught me portion control and brought much-needed balance into my life.

When I quit the gym years ago, I dedicated my exercise time to Ashtanga yoga. Ashtanga yoga is an intense style of yoga that continuously flows from pose to pose, using deep breathing to build strength, flexibility, and endurance. I discuss it in great detail in the next chapter.

Chapter 4
Warning: Ashtanga Yoga Will Change Your Life

Anyone can practice. Young man can practice. Old man can practice. Very old man can practice. Man who is sick, he can practice. Man who doesn't have strength can practice. Except lazy people; lazy people can't practice Ashtanga yoga.
—Sri. K. Pattabhi Jois, Ashtanga Yoga Guru

Out of all the styles of yoga, I recommend Ashtanga more than any other for weight loss and longevity because of its intensity, integrity, and spiritual roots. "Ashtanga" in Sanskrit means "eight limbs." It is a sequence of postures that build upon each other to allow the practitioner to gain incredible strength, flexibility, endurance, and concentration. The sequence is extremely thorough and complete, more than any other style of yoga I have experienced. It touches every part of your body in addition to penetrating the mind and spirit. Ashtanga yoga moves continuously, so you could say there is an element of "cardio" to it, which is helpful for weight loss, as compared to gentle styles of yoga.

Ashtanga yoga is believed to be 5,000 years old and originated in Mysore, India. Sri K. Pattabhi Jois was the Guru of Ashtanga yoga. "Guruji," as his students endearingly called him, taught Ashtanga for 70 years. He introduced it to the West, via Encinitas, California, in 1975. He taught hundreds of thousands of students from all over the world, until he passed in 2009 at the age of 93. He was famous for saying, "Practice and all is coming." I like to think of it as, "Do your practice, all is coming in Divine time." When you show up on your mat, it's an act of showing up for yourself and God. You are deepening your spiritual connection, which in turn will help you in all areas of your life.

I keep this in mind daily when my mind tries to come up with excuses to not practice. I can honestly say I have never had a practice where I didn't feel better at the end of it than I did at the beginning. My yoga practice always makes me feel more alive and connected. It challenges me to grow, on and off the mat, in ways I never expected. I don't know where my life would be today without it.

The Ashtanga system is a set of postures you can memorize and practice anywhere: at home, outside, or in a hotel room. It's nature's perfect exercise, using your own body weight for resistance, which, for most of us, is ample. You will never be bored. I say this with love: Don't expect to be good at it. It's a life-long practice that will keep you inspired and coming back to the mat daily. After all, if you could do everything in your first class, what would be the point? There would be nothing to learn, and it is in the learning where we find growth. I feel Ashtanga was designed to be intentionally unattainable for beginners, with the good intention of helping students grow in their practice. Expect to be challenged, knowing that the practice is here to heal your body and your life. There's a saying in yoga, "Check your ego at the door," and it's true. Yoga is humbling. Many of the students who excel at the practice do so because they are patient and disciplined in their approach to it.

The people I see struggle the most in Ashtanga are actually athletes and marathon runners. They are used to being the "best" at their sport, and then they come to yoga and get frustrated because they don't look good doing it. Remember, no one is judging you but you. The teacher and other students are there to support you, wherever you are in your practice. We all have to start somewhere and build from that point. Honor where you are, be grateful for what your body can do, and don't worry about what it's not ready to do yet. Basically, "Do your best and let go of the rest." Ashtanga yoga teacher Larry Schultz used to say, "Honor your body, but don't be lazy!"

From an exercise physiology viewpoint, I feel Ashtanga yoga is *the* most effective form of exercise in general. It is strength, cardio, flexibility, endurance, all rolled into one practice, PLUS it has meditation and spirituality, if you choose. Traditionally, Ashtanga is practiced six days a week, with Saturdays off. In addition, New and Full Moon days are rest days when you do not practice, as those days can affect the student's energy level. It's also recommended to take rest days during your "ladies' holiday," at least for the first two to three days of your cycle, depending on the intensity. This will help you conserve your energy for your health.

Ashtanga has four series or levels of postures. In the advanced series of Ashtanga, there are several poses in which you press your body up in the air like a gymnast, doing handstands and arm balances. This can take years of practice, so have no fear. I say this not to scare you off, but for you to understand that Ashtanga has an incredible strength component to it. Traditionally, yoga is viewed as more of a stretch and relaxation practice, which it can be if you seek out gentle yoga classes or restorative yoga. My husband likes to joke that when he went to his first yoga class, he thought he was just going to stretch out after doing his "real" weight lifting workout and was surprised how hard it was for him. His comment was, "I had my ass handed to me." However, he fell in love with it immediately, quit lifting weights, enrolled in a yoga teacher training, and was teaching yoga at the same gym within a year.

The Ashtanga system brings balance to both the front and the back of the body. It lengthens your muscles while it strengthens them. For instance, in Down Dog, the quadriceps in the front of your thighs are contracted, getting stronger, while the hamstrings in the back get stretched and lengthened. The muscle groups aren't fighting each other; they are working together as a team. The practice strives to make you equally flexible and strong, not just one or the other. Most forms of cardiovascular exercise, such as running or biking, strengthen the quadriceps while shortening and tightening the hamstrings, creating imbalances in the body that can lead to injuries. If you love to run and cycle, add three days of Ashtanga yoga into your routine to lengthen your muscles and keep your joints flexible. This will help improve your sport performance and prevent injuries.

Ashtanga also helps balance out the right and left side of the body, with the intention of helping them to be equally strong and flexible. If you are right-handed, there's a great chance the right side of your body is stronger and therefore tighter. Ashtanga will help bring these imbalances to the surface to be corrected through the postures and the deep breathing. With a consistent practice, both sides of the body will become more balanced, giving you a sense of freedom in your body.

When I first started yoga over 20 years ago, I had terrible knee pain from running and was worried I needed surgery. I had gone to physical therapy, but nothing seemed to help. My physical therapist said I had run all the miles out of my knees, and she was right. Once I stopped running and started practicing Ashtanga daily, in time the knee pain completely went away. Whenever I try to sneak in a mini jog to get somewhere faster, my knee hurts, as if to say, "Don't you dare go back to your old compulsive cardio ways!" And now, I listen and stop. Ashtanga is a powerful form of physical therapy for your whole body, especially your shoulders, back, knees, and hips. No part of your being will go untouched.

The Ashtanga system includes continuous flowing postures in a vinyasa style of movement, deep breathing, and energy locks, called *bandhas*. These energy locks are located in three places: the throat, low belly (beneath the naval), and perineum, which is located at the floor of the pelvis. The throat lock, *jalandhara bandha*, happens when you tuck your chin towards the jugular notch in your chest. The low belly lock, *uddiyana bandha*, occurs by scooping the space beneath the naval in towards the spine and up, making a lifting motion. The root lock, *mula bandha*, is engaged by lifting the perineum up towards the naval, similar to a Kegel exercise.

Engaging or locking the muscles in these areas, combined with deep breathing, produces an internal heat and a digestive fire called *agni*. Your internal organs get massaged by the locks and purified by the fire, helping you to detoxify, increase your metabolism, and lose weight. You start to move energy from the base of the spine to the crown of the head, helping to remove energetic and emotional blockages that can be keeping you stuck and heavy in your body and your life. The fire also acts as a spiritual fire; it rises into the mind and burns through the fog of illusion and disillusion to give you clear thinking and insight about your life. It releases depression and creates space for joy to enter.

The practice also produces a meditative quality due to the deep rhythmic breathing and memorized sequence. It is calming for the mind and allows you to connect spiritually.

According to yogic philosophy, there are five layers or sheaths *(koshas)* of our being: the physical body, the energy body, the mental body, the wisdom body, and the soul body. Ashtanga yoga cultivates a state of deep devotion and surrender, allowing you to pierce through all the layers to connect to the soul body. This is one of the reasons Ashtanga yoga is a spiritual practice, in addition to an incredible physical experience.

The postures, or "asanas," are only one of the eight limbs of yoga. The other limbs include: moral restraints *(yamas)* self-observations *(niyamas)*, breath control *(pranayama)*, withdrawing the senses inward *(pratyahara)*, concentration *(dharana)*, meditation *(dhyana)*, and bliss *(samadhi)*.

One of the moral restraints is non-harming, *ahimsa*, which is where vegetarianism comes into play in the yogic path. Ahimsa includes remaining conscious that our food choices and actions won't cause harm to other sentient beings and the planet. This helps cultivate a sense of deep compassion for all beings, seeing the Divine in all living creatures, including farm animals and even insects. Consider escorting bugs and spiders outside in a glass jar when possible, instead of killing them, or allowing them to share your space. Remember you are bigger than they are.

I have been teaching Ashtanga since 1997 and have witnessed thousands of people lose weight from this powerful system of yoga, including an 18-year-old girl, Lauren, who lost 100 pounds through practicing Ashtanga yoga daily. Lauren weighed 300 pounds when she began her Ashtanga practice with me and had Polycystic Ovarian Syndrome. However, she didn't let her weight or health condition stop her. She had iron will, showed up to class daily, and was my most dedicated student. As she started to drop the pounds, her self-confidence began to grow, and she began to bloom on the mat and in her life. She is married now with a son and has several degrees.

I also have witnessed people heal anorexia and bulimia, as the practice helps to address the root of their issues, which was usually a lack of self-worth. I've seen people who come to the practice with their head hanging low, barely able to look me in the eye and say hello, begin to transform like butterflies from their daily practice. Their self-esteem improves and their personalities begin to shine and burn through the shyness. Soon they are chatting away with me and other students, making new friends. It's a beautiful thing to witness.

A male friend told me he never excelled in athletics as a child, and that Ashtanga had given him a sense of physical confidence he had never experienced in his youth. This sense of confidence on the mat carried over into his personal life, giving him more self-esteem in his work and relationships.

I've observed the practice help numerous students heal from divorces and watched the practice bring couples together to form life partnerships. When you start practicing yoga daily, you can't live a lie. The truth *(satya)* of your soul comes to the surface, and relationships that aren't aligned with your truth tend to be released from your path. Do not be sad. As the Sufi poet Rumi said in his poem, *The Guesthouse*, "He may be clearing you out for some new delight."

Ask yourself, "Is this relationship giving me energy or draining my energy?" Let go of relationships that aren't serving your highest good to create space for people who will lift you up and support you. Losing the weight of a relationship that is draining the life force out of you and weighing you down energetically and emotionally can definitely make you feel lighter in your being.

This is also true for all the "stuff" in your life. If you find yourself surrounded by clutter in your car and your house, clear out everything that isn't serving your highest good. Go through closets, drawers, bedrooms, the basement and the garage. Give away or sell anything you're not using and don't plan on using anytime soon. In yoga, non-hoarding is called *aparigraha.* This will help you to feel lighter and to think more clearly.

I hope you will give Ashtanga a chance to help you lose weight AND transform your life. Look for an Introduction to Ashtanga class or Mysore style class at a yoga studio in your area. Mysore style is the traditional way of learning the Ashtanga system. The teacher works with each person in the class on a one-on-one basis, customizing the practice to their level and pace. Other practitioners will be in the room with you, working on their own practice at their own pace, while the teacher comes around the room giving hands-on adjustments. Mysore style is the most effective way to learn Ashtanga yoga. It will help you to have more of an internal experience, where you can focus on your breath, memorize the sequence, and become self-sufficient with the practice, as compared to someone always telling you what to do in a led class.

Having a yoga studio and supportive community to go to daily is a wonderful gift and privilege. You can build life-long friendships with your teachers and fellow students and support each other in your practice and personal lives. The people you practice with daily become like your second family or, for some people, like the family they never had.

If you don't have access to a live Ashtanga class, I have resources listed in the Appendix.

Start slowly to build strength and endurance—which happens quickly, especially if you're practicing daily. Even if you can do only five minutes, good for you. The next day, do six minutes, and keep gradually building from there. Don't give up. If you are sore, practice anyway. Yoga isn't like weight lifting, where you take days off in between practices to repair your muscles. In time, with a regular practice of 5-6 days a week, it will become like a second skin. This takes time, dedication, and years of daily practice, but it's worth every ounce of effort and drop of sweat, I promise you. It has been my saving grace on every level. I don't know where I would be without it.

Do your own pilot study and practice Ashtanga yoga six days a week for a month before you make a decision about it. After a month, if you still find it too challenging at this point in your life, experiment with other styles of yoga and teachers to find a class that works for you. Vinyasa yoga also continuously moves and is good for weight loss. It is based on Ashtanga but isn't a set sequence. Make sure your teacher emphasizes deep, rhythmic breathing (*Ujjayi* breath) to help you get the most out of your yoga experience. The deep transformation comes from the breath.

Chapter 5
Walking in Nature Is a Wonder Drug

Walking is magic. Can't recommend it highly enough. The movement, the meditation, the footsteps...this is a primal way to connect with one's deeper self.
—Paul Cole

Walking is my second favorite form of exercise for weight loss and longevity, when done in moderation and in a mindful manner. When possible, walk on asphalt, grass, or sand to reduce the impact on your joints. Walking one to three miles a day is ample, especially if you want to do it for life, so it doesn't wreak havoc on your body. If you're practicing a strong style of yoga daily, a one- to two-mile walk is perfect, so it doesn't hinder your practice by tightening up your quadriceps, hamstrings, groin, hips, and low back.

Keep in mind that excessive cardio can lead to an excessive appetite. Make sure you aren't overdoing exercise in order to eat whatever you want. I had a friend who could barely run on grass anymore because her knees hurt so badly. She wouldn't stop running because she loved ice cream and couldn't quit eating it. This is a common problem for people who spend hours in the gym but never lose weight because they don't want to change their diet. You have to pay attention to what and how much you eat and drink. There's no way of ignoring this important piece of the weight loss journey. Strive to find a loving and healthy balance with food and exercise. Listen to your body's inner wisdom. It knows what it needs and how much.

Like yoga, walking lengthens your muscles and doesn't bulk you out. It also aids your digestion and increases your metabolism. Walk outside, without music, spending time with yourself and the wonders of Mother Nature. Take in the sights and smells and the beauty of your surroundings and make it a moving meditation. The mechanics of walking, combined with the high vibration of nature, can do wonders for the mind. It acts as a natural anti-depressant, easing the mind of stressful thoughts and replacing them with positive thought patterns.

Another way to increase walking in your life—and that isn't as hard on your body as power walking—is what I call "destination" walking. Instead of driving somewhere, make up an excuse to walk. Walk to work, the post office, a friend's house, or a restaurant; no "proper" walking attire and shoes required. Walk around your office, take the stairs instead of the elevator, or park your car far away from the entrance to a building to get more steps into your day.

I walk after lunch to aid my digestion. I walk to my meditation temple and then walk home after I sit, which is only a mile round trip. Nothing much, but I do it daily, so it adds up by the end of the week. I sometimes wear flip-flops because they allow my feet to spread, and it feels more like a walking meditation. I also walk to the grocery store and to the beach for fun. When I have more energy, I also like to put on my "sneaks" and walk around my beautiful neighborhood and on the beach and take in the scenery. These are just a few examples of how you can implement more walking into your daily life.

If you walk the way Europeans walk—as a mode of transportation—and are paying attention to what and how much you eat, excess weight will begin to melt away. Many Europeans who walk everywhere and eat in moderation don't need other forms of exercise. I can see them scoffing, "What is this American gym stuff?" They have balanced lives of moving and eating. In the U.S., we rely way too much on our cars, so make up excuses to walk more and leave your car at home, if possible. Go explore your neighborhood and city by foot and burn some calories while you're at it.

Whatever your exercise of choice, make sure you are exercising smart, meaning the exercise is nurturing your body so you will be able to maintain it for years to come. Think longevity. Make sure it also involves a stretch routine with deep breathing, preferably with your lips sealed. This will increase your flexibility, help prevent injury, and keep you doing your sport of choice longer in life. Stretching is underrated in most fitness routines, because it's not about the "burn." Make a conscious effort to include a stretch routine into your program, even if your fitness instructor doesn't teach it.

Pick activities that aren't going to cause permanent damage as you get older. People will kill themselves with over-exercising to look great in the moment, without thinking of the long-term ramifications of their sport of choice. Men tend do this with weight lifting for a "manly chest," which can cause rotator cuff problems. Women tend to do excess cardio to have a "cute butt," which can cause knee problems. All to achieve some societal standard of what a beautiful body "should" look like. It's not worth it.

Pick forms of exercise that feel right for your body AND, most importantly, put a smile on your face. If you don't enjoy it, you probably won't stick with it long term. Your time is valuable, so you want to pick an activity you enjoy. What you choose to do for your exercise routine today, you want to still be able to do 20+ years from now, throughout the aging process. You want to keep exercising mindfully for life. It's all about finding a balance that works for your body.

One of the many great things about exercise is that it makes your body more metabolically active. Once your exercise session ends, the internal combustion continues to burn calories throughout your day while you're sitting at your desk, eating a meal, and even while you're sleeping. It's a beautiful thing. Exercising is extremely helpful in the weight loss process. Make it a part of your daily life. For weight loss, exercise a minimum of 30 minutes a day, 7 days a week, and longer when you have the time and energy. The key is to move every day. Establish exercise as a part of your daily routine. It is better to exercise a little bit every day than two hours at a time, three days a week. Focus on the frequency of your exercise program and not just the duration. Exercising daily will keep your metabolism fired up on a regular basis and help your mind to feel happy.

Exercise is also helpful for your digestion and regular bowel movements. You want to make sure you are having a least one bowel movement a day to keep your colon healthy. Drink a large glass of water first thing when you get up each morning to stimulate your bowels. Continue to focus on drinking water instead of caffeine throughout your day so your colon doesn't get dehydrated, which can lead to constipation, blockages, and hard stools. Eating a plant-based diet high in fiber will help clear out your colon on a daily basis. If your bowels need assistance, try Organic Smooth Move Herbal Tea, by Traditional Medicinals Teas. You can also take a magnesium citrate supplement, without the calcium. Magnesium relaxes the muscles in the intestines and it also attracts water, which will soften your stools. If you have kidney disease, however, you may have excess magnesium, so don't take it as a supplement. Take a non-dairy probiotic daily to keep your gut populated with healthy bacteria.

I'm also a proponent of monthly colonics (colon hydrotherapy), which is a personal choice for you to make. Your colon (large intestine) is about five feet long. If you have regular bowel movements, it's probably only pushing out last night's meal and not the years of stool build-up that can line the intestinal wall. Even if you are regular, it's sci-fi what still remains in the colon. It's important to get this putrefied food out of your colon so it doesn't become toxic and lead to disease in the body. I resisted colonics for a long time, but once I started getting them, I understood their value in improving health and preventing disease. My husband, who has had cancer, is a huge fan of them. He says, "If your septic system is backed up, your house is going to smell." This can lead to health and skin problems and chronic bad breath.

My colonic therapist calls the colon the "second brain." He works with people who are both at their ideal weight and overweight. He also treats people with allergies, digestion problems, cancer, Crohn's disease, and skin issues such as eczema and acne. Look for a licensed colonic therapist in your area, ask for referrals from friends, and read reviews before making an appointment.

MIND & SPIRIT

Chapter 6
Prayer Is Talking to God as a Best Friend

Prayer is the conduit for miracles.
—A Course in Miracles

If someone asked me who my best friend was, I would happily say, "God." My friends have come and gone through the years, but God has always been by my side. I grew up going to church with my family, but it was a Sunday-only experience, like it is for many people. We didn't talk about God at home, but for as long as I can remember, I would talk to God as I would my best friend.

Fast forward 40 years, and I'm still chatting away with God, out loud, wherever I go: at my altar, in my car, at my desk, and before I embark on a work or social event, asking to be guided and giving thanks. Shortly after I met my husband in Los Angeles, we were walking through the grocery store aisle, and he asked me who I was talking to. I said, "God and Jesus." He never asked again.

Sometimes I worry I am boring God with the insignificant details of my life and will start my prayers off with, "Dear God, I know this may sound trivial, but..." Then I realize, nothing is too mundane or profound for the Creator of the Universe.

God is there for you, too, on a minute-to-minute basis, waiting to connect with you. I suggest you pray to God about

EVERYTHING. Make this a daily practice in opening the lines of communication between you and the Divine and see what starts to happen in your life. Ask for your relationship with food to be healed. Ask for help to heal any root issues within yourself that are triggering you to overeat. Ask for the strength and courage to heal food addictions and any other unhealthy addictions in your life. Pray for discipline in your food choices and for the strong will to exercise daily. Pray to meet like-minded people and to be guided to groups who can support you in living a healthy lifestyle and lift you up to be your best self. Pray to love and accept yourself as God loves and accepts you, unconditionally. Nourish your relationship with God on a daily basis, letting God know you are serious about cultivating a relationship.

Ask for your life purpose to be revealed and to have passion about your earthly assignment. When people are aligned with their soul's calling, they are happier, more focused, and less depressed. For many, weight loss happens naturally when they are in the space of feeling fulfilled with their purpose and having a sense of community in their lives. I see a lot of people gain weight who are miserable at their jobs. I've been there.

When you bound out of bed each day, knowing you are part of a bigger plan that is greater than yourself, the focus becomes more about "we" and not just "me." God created you with a unique set of talents and gifts that only YOU can offer in that certain special way. Your gifts can easily help to enrich the lives of humans, animals, and the environment. Pray to be of service and to fulfill your destiny. Know that your presence on the planet at this moment in time is intentional and that you matter. The world needs you.

Prayer is often described as "telephoning God," meaning you are the one making the call and talking to God. Pray for clarity about work, relationships, to be more patient, to control anger…whatever you are feeling. Just get it all out of you so those feelings aren't harboring inside of you, keeping you energetically stuck and physically heavy. Know that God is hearing you, whether you see immediate results or not. Ask for signs of synchronicity in your life and pay attention to who is standing next to you in line at the grocery store or the post office.

I acquired one of my cats years ago because I was standing in line at Long's Drugs store, and a man overheard a conversation I was having with the cashier. He said, "Do you want another cat?" It turned out an abandoned cat had been living in his backyard and needed a forever home. Lucky me! Adopting Natasha was one of the most heartfelt experiences of my life.

You just never know who or what God may use to deliver a message to you: a stranger, a family member, a friend, a co-worker, an email, a phone call, or a letter. The ways that answers can come are infinite, so be aware and look for signs. Pay attention to the unseen world, beyond your physical eyes. Look for the magic in ordinary events. If you believe in angels, invoke them into your life and talk to them as well. ASK THEM TO HELP YOU.

As you feel more connected in your relationship with God and the spiritual realm, you will begin to feel a sense of interconnectedness and oneness with all life. One of the common reasons people overeat is due to feelings of loneliness. Prayer and meditation are constant reminders that you always have a spiritual companion in life and are never alone. I have always secretly hoped to be interviewed by Oprah, so she could ask me her signature question, "What do you know for sure?" I would smile, tear up, and reply, "We are never alone."

Chapter 7
Meditation Is God Calling You

Meditation is like giving a hug to ourselves, getting in touch with that awesome reality in us. While meditating we feel a deep sense of intimacy with God, a love that is inexplicable.
—Paramahansa Yogananda

One of the biggest reasons people overeat is stress. Meditation *(dhyana)* acts as a tool to remove stressful thoughts of anxiety and depression and replace them with thoughts of clarity and hope. Meditation reminds the mind that everything is going to be okay.

The mind is full of incessant thoughts that keep us in a constant state of "wanting." *I want a doughnut, a cup of coffee, a slice of pizza, a glass of wine, a new pair of shoes, and of course, sex!* The list is endless. Pretty soon our minds are like a pinball machine, pinging bells in our head for every whimsical desire. The mind is like a small child, getting upset when it doesn't get what it wants, when it wants it. This is why we need to establish mental discipline to help us differentiate between impulsive wants and basic needs, especially when it comes to food and true physiological hunger.

The greatest gift for discernment I have ever received is the practice of meditation. Meditation is quieting our thoughts so we can connect to the voice of our soul and to God. Think of meditation as God telephoning you, and you sitting back and listening. Visualize a wire of electricity between your mind and

God. The static on the line is the thousands of thoughts and desires you have each day. Meditation helps reduce the static on the line so you can have a clearer connection with God. Meditation is different from prayer, because you are being receptive and listening instead of being proactive and talking. However, at some point in your meditation, you may want to have an internal dialogue in which you ask for guidance and then sit back and listen. No rules; just do what comes naturally. This is a powerful practice of surrendering to the Divine *(Ishvara Pranidhana.)*

Meditation also brings discipline into the mind so you are better able to control your cravings and emotions and achieve your life goals. Meditation does this by aligning your mind with Divine Mind, Universal Intelligence, or God's Mind—whatever name you want to give it. When your mind is aligned and filled with Divine source energy, your unhealthy habits will lose their power over you, as happens in yoga. You will have more self-discipline in all areas of your life. Why is this so?

The more time you spend in silence with God, the more your mind will become fulfilled from the inside out, and the more you will notice a shift in your consciousness. Your mind will be, for a lack of better word, "super" charged with Divine energy, filled with more thoughts from your Higher Self than your lower, weaker self. You will begin to make healthier and more conscious choices, such as eating less meat and quitting alcohol. The need to self-destruct will diminish, because those incessant desires are now being replaced by the still small voice of your soul, who always wants the best for you.

As you spend more time in stillness, you will begin to love and accept yourself as God loves you—unconditionally. This feeling of unconditional love will become more pervasive than the self-limiting thoughts, helping you to release the need to binge on food or other external substances. When you feel better about yourself, there will be less tendency to desecrate your body temple.

Let me give you an example—one I'm not proud of by any means. When I was in my 20s, I smoked when I drank alcohol. "I'm a social smoker," was my excuse. One Halloween, my girlfriend had come to visit me in Kansas City. We were dressed in our 70s attire, ready to party for the night. We started off with drinks at my apartment, but when I went to light up a cigarette, it was as if a force field came down between me and the cigarette, and it tasted horrible, like dirt. But I was determined to smoke, so I took another drag. It tasted even worse. I thought, "What is going on?"

I was new to yoga and meditation at the time. But now, 20 years later, my interpretation of the event is that my Higher Self was putting the kibosh on my nasty little habit. I'm upset with myself for smoking in the first place, but that was my consciousness at that time of my life. As the saying goes, "When you know better, you do better." My smoking days ended that night, and meditation and yoga can do the same thing for you when it comes to overeating.

This example is just one of the many reasons why it is imperative to make daily meditation a part of your life, no matter what your mind conjures up for an excuse. Unfortunately, the ego mind has a strong pattern of keeping us incessantly busy, saying we don't have time for meditation...which is like saying we don't have time for God. The mind will do anything to sabotage us from connecting to God, such as focusing on work, emailing, texting, exercising, watching TV, car-pooling kids, grocery shopping, cooking, and pets…not to mention a full-time job. Trust me, I understand all of these activities can EASILY consume a day. The bottom line is that it comes down to prioritizing, combined with time management, to make your relationship with God a top priority in your life.

The irony of blowing off meditation is that we think we are too busy with all the wonderful gifts God has given us, so we forget to give back to the Giver of the gifts. Meditation allows us time to give back to God by focusing on our inward connection. We are showing our love and appreciation for God and for all the blessings in our lives. Like any relationship, you have to nurture it to grow. By making God a priority in our lives, we are showing God we want to have a relationship and that we care. The great yogi Paramahansa Yogananda used to say, "Everything else in your life can wait, but your search for God cannot wait."

If you think about it, all these things you think you are too "busy" with to meditate are not going with you when you leave the physical body. The one thing that is going with you is your connection to God. The body isn't coming with you, your friends and family are not coming with you, your bed isn't coming with you, your snacks aren't coming with you, and your phones and computers aren't coming with you. Put the Divine first in your life and nurture THE most important relationship every day and not just on one day a week or on holidays. Many times, we think God has abandoned us, but if we are honest with ourselves, we are the ones abandoning God. God is always there for us. The question is, "Are we making the effort to show up for God?" Meditation is one of the best ways to spend time with God and to keep the lines of communication flowing in both directions, every morning and every night.

Practice meditation first thing in the morning and right before bed, after you wash your face. This will help you be more alert for your sit. Set up a small sacred space in a room in your house, a corner of a room, or even in a closet. Any space where you can have quiet time alone is perfect. Set up an altar on a small table or wooden box and put a colorful piece of fabric over it. Place a candle in the middle of the altar and add items to it that represent your connection to Spirit, such as a photo of Jesus or a statue of Buddha, Ganesha, or whoever speaks to your soul. You can also add a photograph of a relative or a pet who has made their earthly transition, to remind you of your eternal bond together.

After you have established your sacred space, place a cushion in front of your altar and sit in an upright seated position, with a straight spine. If you are brand new to meditation, you may need to prop your back up against a wall for support. In time, the muscles aligning your spine will get stronger, and you will be able to sit without the wall.

Place your hands on your legs, way up by your hip bones, with the palms up. This will help keep the spine straight so the energy can flow without being obstructed by a rounded back. Take five deep, cleansing breaths, inhaling through the nose and exhaling out through either the nose or mouth. This will help you release tension, emotions, and life experiences that aren't serving your highest good. The breaths will also quiet the mind chatter and calm your nervous system, helping you to release the events of the day so you can focus in the present moment.

Next, close the eyes and focus the internal between your eyebrows. In yoga, this is know spiritual third eye, or seat of concentration. F point gives your mind a single gazing point, the mind still and the eyes from dropping. A meditation, if the eyes feel heavy and sleepy, "flip" them right back up to this point and concentrate deeply into the third eye. Think of this spiritual eye as a portal, connecting you inward to your soul and to God.

As you focus the internal gaze to the point between your eyebrows, begin breathing naturally through the nose, with lips sealed. Inhale and exhale through the nose without control or sound. Next, add a silent mantra to match your breath. "Mantra" is a Sanskrit word that means "instrument for the mind" and is a word, statement, or sound that you repeat silently or out loud. A mantra gives the mind something to concentrate on during the meditation session.

The first mantra ever given to me was from a hip Presbyterian Minister, Ann, whom I met on a yoga retreat at Mount Madonna ashram on top of a mountain in California. (How's *that* for hip?) I asked Pastor Ann, "What do you think is the best way to know God?" and then listed off a few of my favorite ways, such as yoga, prayer, and reading spiritual texts. Without delay, she said, "Hands down, meditation." She then gave me the mantra, "Be Still and Know," telling me to inhale while silently repeating "Be Still" and exhale while silently repeating "and Know." This mantra is from Psalm 46:10, "Be still and know that I am God." I like to interpret it as if God is saying to my chatter-filled mind, "Be still and know that I am taking care of all your needs. Surrender them to me. P.S I love you."

...ll and know" works like a charm on the mind. It acts ...ixir, canceling out fear-based thoughts such as doubt, ...y, anger, and anxiety. It is a friendly reminder that there is ...oving God watching over you, guiding every area of your ...ife. Vietnamese Zen Master Thich Nhat Hanh wrote a book entitled *Be Still and Know*, teaching this universal mantra as well.

With every round of this mantra, you are continuously reminded that God is your constant co-pilot throughout life, navigating you to the right resources, people, places, and experiences to help you fulfill your destiny. Prayer and meditation help us to discern when it's time to take action in our lives and when it's time to wait and surrender. It takes the pressure off of having to know and do everything by yourself, because you know you have spiritual help available— especially if you're asking for it and paying attention for the answers.

Once you've established your meditation area and mantra, I suggest sitting five minutes every morning upon awakening and five minutes before going to bed. Yes, you will have to get up earlier, but it will be worth it. It seems that "sleep" is the number one excuse among my students for not meditating. People LOVE their sleep...so, just go to bed five minutes earlier the night before. Problem solved.

Human beings tend to want to do anything to avoid spending time in silence with their thoughts and feelings. They would rather run miles, swim laps, lift weights, or do handstands for an hour than sit for five minutes in silence with themselves. The mind is the hardest muscle to train, but it is the most important one, because it is the decision maker in your life. If your mind is always aligned with high adrenaline, nonstop activity and is dosed with caffeine, there will be no space for God to speak to you nor for you to hear the voice of your soul. Don't run or hide from yourself. "Busyness" can be a disease if you're not conscious of its hold on your life. There's a Zen proverb that says, "To be truly hard and strong, one must be pliable and soft." Meditation and yoga can help you find balance between activity and rest, and effort and surrender.

If you sit five minutes in the morning and five minutes before bed, this equals ten minutes a day or 70 minutes a week. It's amazing how just five minutes of stillness can accumulate by the end of the week. It's just a matter of sitting yourself down on the cushion. As yoga teacher Rolf Gates says in his book *Meditations from the Mat*, "Staple butt to cushion."

If five minutes is too long, start with two minutes and build your way up, adding one minute each day. Your mind is going to wander in the beginning, like a monkey swinging from thought to thought, not wanting to be still. Have no judgment if this happens. It's normal. After all, this is the nature of the mind. It likes to think.

If your mind starts making a shopping list or thinking about what you're going to eat for your next meal, acknowledge these thoughts and then let them go, knowing you have the rest of the day to address them. Return to your mantra to tether the mind into stillness. This sacred time is for you to have a recess from thinking and to experience stillness in a waking state. In time, you are going to experience longer gaps in between your thoughts. I like to think of it like Morse code: thought, thought, gap, thought, gap, thought, gaaaaaaaaaap. With enough daily practice, your mind will slip into the gaps between your thoughts, where you can experience peace and stillness. Sometimes, when I am praying before bed, my mind will drift into a gap instead. I get excited, because I can tell my mind wants me to meditate, not talk. I consider this progress.

After your first week of meditating, I suggest increasing your meditation time to ten minutes every morning and ten minutes every night. Do that for a week. Then, continue to increase your time each week, in increments of 1-5 minutes, until you have reached 20 minutes in the morning and 20 minutes at night. At any point during your meditation, you can let go of the mantra and speak to God inwardly from the language of your heart and then sit back and listen. Here are some examples: "What do you want me to know?" and "How can I serve?"

Meditation will help you fill up spiritually, instead of stuffing your feelings with food. When your mind is aligned with Divine Mind, your thoughts will be more positive and loving towards yourself and others. The self-loathing thought patterns that contributed to your weight gain cannot help you lose the weight. *A Course in Miracles* would say that you need a "a shift in perception," which is the definition of a miracle. Meditation can give you this shift in perception, which can help you lose weight permanently.

Here is a list of suggested mantras for meditation. Try a new one out each week and see which one resonates with you:

Inhale	Exhale
Be Still	And know
I Am	At Peace
Let Go	Let God
I Am	Divine Love
Om (sound of the Universe)	Peace
Om	Spirit or Christ or God

Meditation Summary

- Create an altar in a quiet corner in yo
- Sit with a straight spine in a comforta
  position. Sit on a pillow to elevate hips, if needed.
- Use a wall if your spine needs support.
- Rest hands on the backs of the knees or up by the hips,
  palms up.
- Focus internal gaze, with eyes closed, on the point
  between the eyebrows.
- Pick a mantra and repeat the words silently and
  frequently.
- Practice every morning and every night, without
  judgment of your thoughts.
- Begin with five minutes in the morning and five
  minutes before you go to bed.
- Increase in increments of 1-5 minutes weekly, until you
  reach 20 minutes.
- With regular practice, the thoughts will subside, and
  you will slip into the gap between your thoughts and
  experience the stillness of your soul.

You can also use a meditation app, such as Insight Timer,
to track your meditations and your progress.

Chapter 8
Journaling Is Being Pen Pals with the Universe

The starting point of discovering who you are, your gifts, your talents, your dreams, is being comfortable with yourself. Spend time alone. Write in a journal.
—Robin S. Sharman

Beginning in grade school, I started writing in my diary. I realize now that "Dear Diary" was synonymous with "Dear God." I would share my thoughts and feelings, helping me to clear my mind and vent my perceived adolescent problems.

When I was older, I started journaling daily to help me heal the past and to put out prayers to the Universe for my future. Through the years I accumulated a collection of over 40 journals, filled with dreams, dramas, old boyfriends, and letters to God. As in prayer, I expressed my thoughts, fears, and desires, but through the written word. My journals supported me like trusted friends enduring life's challenges and celebrations together. Through the years, I found solace in my journaling "alone" time, along with a good cup of tea.

I recently let go of my lifetime journal collection in preparing for my move from Kansas City, Missouri, to Encinitas, California. I had moved my journals from location to location for years, and they were just sitting stagnant in my basement. Some of them were too tragic to even read. Who was that poor girl? From a Feng Shui perspective, I decided they were stagnant energy and not serving me anymore. I was hoping the symbolism of shredding them and starting fresh with a new journal would help me release the past and open up to a new future. I think it might have worked, because I am now living my dream of being a writer and life coach, living by the ocean. I'm convinced journaling and a lot of praying got me here. Thanks God.

I suggest you get a beautiful journal or make your own, something that is pretty and inspires you to open it on a daily basis. Julia Cameron, author of *The Artist's Way,* encourages people to write their Artist Pages every day. Just sit down and start writing. You may think you don't have anything to say, and out might come a flood of emotions, thoughts and feelings, which is therapeutic and healing for your soul. You learn a lot about yourself when you start putting it down in writing. I suggest you do this practice of self-study *(swadhyaya)* daily and see what comes up for you. I think you will be pleasantly surprised how much you have to say, without really thinking about it. Write until you can't write anymore. Clear the channels of blocked emotions through the power of your pen.

You can also record a food diary to help you be more aware of exactly what you are eating and drinking and how much. This will serve as a reference point for your diet. This isn't an exercise in punishment or guilt, but a practice in awareness. We have a tendency to think some of our favorite foods and beverages are calorie-free because of our deep love for them...like my mochas and scones. Weigh yourself once a week and record it in your journal as well. You can also use phone applications, like LOSE IT or FIT BIT to track your food and exercise.

Once you have your food diary in place, analyze it to see what simple changes you could make in your diet to improve your health and lose weight. A friend cut soda from his diet, and he lost 10 pounds from that one simple change. For you, it might be cutting back on eating meat, eliminating dairy or fast food, eating fewer potato chips, or going out to eat less often. The next week, make another diet modification that is for your highest good, like bringing your lunch to work. Then keep building from there until you start to see some noticeable changes in your body and on the scale.

If you tend to overeat, binge, or have a compulsion for unhealthy foods, write down what you are FEELING before you binge (or afterwards, if it's already occurred). This exercise will help you uncover the core belief you are experiencing and help you shift it. This can potentially ward off future binges. Are you feeling lonely, sad, unworthy, unloved? Why? What are these emotions trying to tell you? Write it all out. Our minds can be our worst enemy and our best friend, all in a five-minute time period. Your thoughts are not facts. They are just thoughts, and you have the power to shift limiting beliefs to positive ones, such as transforming "I'm not worthy," to, "I am worthy and deserving of my heart's desires." You always have a choice.

To help stave off this love-hate relationship with yourself, start journaling daily. Get everything out on paper and don't hold back. This isn't an exercise about playing it safe or being polite. If you're angry, write it down and don't feel guilty about it. If you're feeling "less than" or ignored by someone in your life, write it down. If you're feeling grateful, write it down. Keep it real and don't censor a thing. You want these emotions out of you, so they don't keep you hostage in your life and impact your food choices and weight.

At the end of the day, write down a minimum of three things you are grateful for in your life, beginning with yourself. The rest can be simple: I am grateful for a healthy body, a sunny day, a roof over my head, a comfortable bed, or a warm shower. If you've ever spent time in a third world country, you know that many of the things we take for granted are considered a privilege in other parts of the world. I've been to India twice and witnessed the extreme poverty, which has made me grateful to have life's basic necessities.

Even on a seemingly less-than-stellar day, writing down a few positive reminders can help give you an attitude of gratitude, which is a positive way to go to bed. Health is always an important one to remember. In time, you'll come to recognize the blessings in your day on a regular basis and will begin to attract more of them into your life.

Chapter 9
Affirmations: Love Yourself Lean

Love yourself first and everything else will fall into line.
You really have to love yourself to get anything done in this
world.
—Lucille Ball

Affirmations are another powerful tool to help you lose weight. My first exposure to using words to create my life was in a book called *The Wisdom of Florence Scovel Shinn,* by Florence Scovel Shinn. It's a life-changer. I have probably read it ten times and can never get enough of Florence's wisdom.

Flo, as I like to call her, was an artist and metaphysician living in New York City in the early 1900s. She said, "Your word is your wand or your sword. You are either creating or destroying by the power of your tongue."

If people were having problems in their life, they would go to Flo to get a "treatment" for their minds. This was called a "truth statement." Florence encouraged people to demand the "Divine Design" of their lives, where all conditions were permanently perfect: perfect health, perfect love, perfect work, perfect home, and perfect money. According to Flo, the Divine Design for your life is God's will for your life. You aren't trying to manifest something that isn't for your highest good and the highest good of all involved.

Here's an example: Sometimes what you want in life isn't in your best interest, but you REALLY want it anyway. Think about your dating history here. Did you ever swoon over someone who ignored you, didn't treat you well, or broke your heart? Even though it felt devastating in the moment, hopefully you came to realize why it didn't work out with that person and that God had someone better suited for you down the timeline of your life. This is an example of the divine plan of your life for "perfect love."

Here is a Flo-ism for the divine plan of your life: "I give thanks for the divine plan of my life where ALL conditions are permanently perfect."

I suggest saying this statement enthusiastically throughout the day to remind yourself that there is a divine plan for every area of your life, including perfect health and the right weight for your body. You want to align your words and thoughts with this plan, so they can intersect.

I heard Life Coach Martha Beck speak about affirmations; she said we need to use both sides of the brain when saying them. When you say them without feeling, you are only using the left side of your brain, the intellectual side. You need the right, creative side of your brain to add feelings and emotions to your affirmations. You will increase the vibration of your words and they will take flight like an airplane, rather than being lifeless sounds lying low to the ground. As your enthusiastic words are lifted, your vibration increases and you begin to attract, like a magnet, that which is yours by divine right. If the divine plan for your life is on a high vibration but your vibration is low, the two can't connect. They are like two airplanes passing over each other in the night—good for airplanes, but not for your divine plan. You need your vibration to be HIGH, so you can align, or politely collide, with the divine plan of your life. If your vibe is down in the dumps and negative, there's less chance you will connect with your plan.

So instead of just saying monotone affirmations like an automaton, put some burning zeal behind them and maybe add a little cheerleading shout or arm gesture to really tell the universe you are serious. "I love my body and my body loves me!" Say it repeatedly throughout your day while looking in the mirror, until you believe the words to be true, even if you have to fake it to make it. Keep making positive declarations about your body, creating an imprint into your consciousness until the affirmations become your prevalent thoughts.

You want to spend MORE time throughout your day speaking and feeling what you *do* want in your life than dwelling on what you don't. If your mind is more focused on negativity, such as "I am fat and lazy," you could easily attract more of that into your life. You want to shift your vibration from overweight and depressed to lean and happy. "I am the perfect weight now." Speak your truth *(satya)* about what you want for your body and your life.

Louise Hay, the founder of Hay House Publishing and author of the bestselling book *You Can Heal Your Life*, was also inspired by Florence's work. Louise was an abused child who didn't graduate from high school. She left home at age fifteen. She attributes her success both personally and professionally to the use of affirmations. In *You Can Heal Your Life*, she promotes the use of affirmations to shift old thought patterns and replace them with new, positive ones. Since most of your negative habitual thoughts, such as "I'm not good enough," began in early childhood, it's important for you to take an inventory of your life to assess what healing still needs to occur.

This isn't intended to blame your parents for what you perceive they did and didn't do, but to have awareness of the emotional influences in your life and how they are impacting you in the present. We need to make peace with the fact that our parents were doing the best they could with the consciousness they had at that time in their lives. We also need to remember they were once young children and had their own set of parental issues instilled in them as well. This isn't to excuse abusive behavior, but to help you understand your parents better so you can live freely in the present.

Vying for a parent's approval year after year and never getting it can leave you feeling "less than" and drained. Let go of trying to please your parents or anyone else in your life. I often wonder if this "need for approval" is really a compassionate lesson from the Universe in disguise to teach us to approve of ourselves. The only approval you need is from God, and God gave it to you the day you were born. The love and acceptance you didn't receive as a child can be given to you in any moment by yourself and by God.

It can be a life-long process of letting go of resentment and unforgiveness. This is a deep healing on your part. It takes courage and a commitment of self-study in order to get to the root of these toxic emotions and release them for good. Prayer, meditation, journaling, affirmations, and yoga can all be helpful in this process, in addition to professional therapy if needed.

Affirmation for forgiveness: "I am willing to love and forgive everyone, including myself." —Louise Hay

If you don't release resentment and unforgiveness, they can keep you stuck in the past and heavy in your body. They can also manifest as disease and hinder your evolution as a soul. These energies can keep you blocked from attracting all the good, love, and abundance life has to offer you. I know it's not easy, but it's imperative for you to lose these emotions so you can also lose the excess weight once and for all. Don't abuse your body for something someone did to you in the past. Nurture, honor, and love your body for the beautiful temple it is to your soul. As my life coach, Dr. Eve Agee, says, "My body is a miracle. My body supports me."

Affirmations help eject the old, negative, and fear-based tapes in your head and replace them with new, positive tapes filled with statements of self-love and acceptance. Repeat this affirmation several times each day: "I deeply and completely love and accept myself." Say it when you look at yourself in the mirror, throughout your day, and especially when you step on the scale.

You may feel some resistance to these words initially, but in time you will begin to embrace yourself for who you are in this moment—not who you will be when you lose 20 pounds, get a new job, get married, or move to a new city. The point of acceptance is *now*, not later. Keep nourishing yourself with positive words of praise and acceptance. Be your own best friend and #1 fan. If saying mean things to yourself hasn't produced the results you desire in your life, it's time to take a more loving approach.

The words "I AM" represents your Higher Self *(Atman)*. You want to use these words in a positive context. Be careful not use them in a negative way such as, "I am a loser." This is like shooting daggers into your soul. You don't want to defame your beautiful "I AM" Self, because your body and life are listening. Make it a daily practice to choose your thoughts and words wisely. Keep loving yourself lean to help you achieve your weight loss goals.

There is great power in saying affirmations with conviction and positive emotions behind them. They truly can produce miracles in your life, sometimes even the same day. Say them first thing upon awakening, in the shower, while walking outside in nature, in your car on your way to work, and before you go to bed. You can never say them too often, especially when you're trying to change a life-long pattern of negative self-talk. It's going to take several repetitions to eliminate the old imprints in your mind, so don't give up. Louise Hay refers to it as "weight lifting for the mind." Keep saying affirmations to promote a shift in consciousness to help you love and accept yourself unconditionally.

I believe self-love is the greatest form of weight loss. It's time to love yourself like you've loved no other. This love will shift your energy field and your relationship with your body and food. When you love and respect yourself, you will want to take better care of yourself, which will help you lose weight. In addition, the more you love yourself, the more love you will attract into your life, including friendships, family, community, and partnerships. Be a love magnet!

FOOD

Chapter 10
A Vegan Diet Is a Win for Humans, Animals, and the Planet

Nothing will benefit human health and increase the chances for survival of life on earth as much as the evolution to a vegetarian diet.
—Albert Einstein.

Before now, you were probably thinking, "This is the first weight loss book that doesn't talk about food." That's not my intention. Food, like politics and religion, is a personal choice. It is also fuel for your body temple. Trying to get someone to shift their food patterns can be as traumatizing as taking away a Linus blanket or as enlightening as a spiritual awakening. I've seen both sides of the coin, from witnessing grown adults having meltdowns over food attachments, to people seeing the light and willingly making more conscious food choices. I held off on discussing food for two main reasons:

1. If I had started the book with what I thought you should eat, you might have stopped reading by now—unless I had said you could eat whatever you wanted. Then I would be your new best friend. No one wants to be told what they can and cannot eat, and I certainly don't enjoy being the food police.

2. I feel the mind/body/spirit connection needs to be addressed first in order for you to be successful in managing your weight for life. Without this imperative

connection, there's a great chance your weight and food will always be a challenge for you.

You might have guessed by now that I'm going to suggest you eat plants, and lots of them! A vegan, plant-based diet is optimal for weight loss, weight management, disease prevention and, in many cases, disease reversal.

I've been vegan since 2002 and feel it was the best choice I ever made for my health, in addition to helping animals and the environment. Ten BILLION farm animals are killed each year in the U.S alone for food, and this doesn't include fish. One million chickens are consumed every hour. This is a cruel tragedy that doesn't have to happen. There are thousands of delicious plant-based food options available for consumption.

Animal agriculture is also taking its toll on the planet, with high greenhouse gas emissions and the use of a tremendous amount of land and water. Rainforests in the Amazon are being cut down to grow soybeans to feed farm animals instead of feeding starving people. As the human population grows, our resources are being depleted. This won't be sustainable in years to come. The movie *Cowspiracy* goes into great detail about this issue and is available on Netflix.

According to National Geographic, it takes 1,800 gallons of water to produce one pound of beef, 468 gallons for a pound of chicken, 576 gallons for a pound of pork, and 880 gallons for a single gallon of milk. In a time of great drought, these numbers are even more significant.
(http://environment.nationalgeographic.com/environment/freshwater/embed ded-water/)

A vegan diet is a win-win-win for humans, animals, and the environment. No one has to suffer or be killed for food. It's a beautiful way to take your yoga practice off the mat by practicing *ahimsa* (non-harming) towards all beings and Mother Earth. Here is how I became vegetarian and then vegan. I hope my story will help inspire you.

Chapter 11
My Vegetarian Awakening Thanks to Guru Samantha the Cat

If slaughter houses had glass walls, everyone would be vegetarian.
—Paul McCartney

My family ate meat every night as far back as I can remember. It was never a consideration not to eat it. One night when I was in the first grade, I was asked to take a last bite of roast before I got up from the table. I was a picky eater at the time, so my parents were trying to get me to eat anything other than my favorite food group: sugar. I put the bite of roast in my mouth and just sat there, unable to swallow. I felt like my soul was screaming, "Don't do it!" Unfortunately, I did, and immediately regretted it. I felt physically ill.

A few hours later, while my mom was reading me the book *Curious George the Monkey,* I jumped off the bed and started vomiting all the way to the bathroom. I think George felt my angst. Thank goodness the message became loud and clear to my parents: "Your daughter doesn't want to eat beef." So every Sunday, when the family would have hamburger night, my mom would give me a can of Spaghetti-O's minus the meatballs, and my soul was happy again.

I wish I could say I gave up eating all meat at an early age, but, sadly, I didn't. I always had a strong affinity towards animals, even stuffed ones, and considered them my friends. I had no idea how meat got to my plate, except probably thinking it magically appeared via the grocery store. If someone had told me the truth, I'm sure I would have had a melt-down. I remember being 4-years old standing next to my mom at a butcher shop and feeling nauseated, now I understand why.

In my early 30s I was still eating a little seafood until our family cat, Samantha, woke me up. Samantha lived to be 22 years old, without a single health problem, until she suddenly came down with kidney failure. I remember my mom calling me to tell me that something was wrong with Samantha. I drove three hours to my hometown to find my childhood cat walking sideways, like she was drunk. Her kidneys were toxic, and she was losing bodily functions. I immediately told my mom we needed to put her out of her misery first thing the next morning.

That night, I wrote Samantha a long letter, stating how much I loved her and how much she had touched my life from the ages of 9 to 31. I was devastated, but I knew I needed to let her go. She was clearly suffering and ready to pass. I spent the night on the kitchen floor with her, and the next morning my mom and I took her to the vet.

I decided it was my responsibility as her human to hold her during the euthanasia process, so I would be the last face she saw in her lifetime. As I held her frail body, the vet gracefully injected her, allowing her to pass from this life to more life. I felt her soul being released. She was free. I was left holding an empty shell of what use to house the soul of my beloved pet. In that instant, the message was clear to me: "ALL animals have souls." I had no right eating any of them. Samantha sent me this message loud and clear. I will always be grateful for this awakening.

If you've ever had to put a pet to sleep, you can relate to my story. Our beautiful companion animals bring us unconditional love and companionship like no other human being. They are our best friends in every sense of the word and stick by us through all of life's ups and downs. They forgive us when we are at our worst, and love us when we don't love ourselves. We know they feel love, compassion, pain, and suffering, just like humans. We see it, we feel it, and we know it to be true in our souls.

However, throughout human history, we divided animals into two groups: companion animals, such as cats and dogs, and food animals, such as cows, pigs, and chickens. We decided companion animals were deserving of love, compassion, and fluffy beds inside the house, but food animals were to be disregarded as if they didn't feel pain, suffering, love, and compassion. It sounds like survival of the cutest.

If you spend time around farm animals, you can see the light in their eyes and the joy in their personalities as they frolic together. They have feelings. They have families, babies, and friends. They enjoy being petted and loved, just like cats and dogs do. I have rested my head on the bellies of pigs and felt the warmth of their skin on my face. They are loving, sweet, and intelligent. I pray for the day humans can extend the love and compassion they have for their pets to all animals, fish, birds, and insects. Reverence for all life forms.

If you've witnessed footage of factory farms or slaughterhouses, it becomes clear very quickly that the final moments of a farm animal's life, even if it's "local," "organic," "free range," or "grass fed," can be filled with fear, suffering, and betrayal by their humans. Animals are smart. They sense fear, and this energy is felt by the surrounding herd. They know what is happening to them.

Reverend Michael Beckwith of Agape church in Los Angeles, who was in the movie *The Secret*, said the following about becoming vegetarian: "Over 30 years ago before I started Agape in the '70s, I became a vegetarian because I was very sensitive to the violence that was happening to the animals. I actually was having a meal and I became very sensitive to the fear that was in the food that I was eating and I became a vegetarian on the spot."

What is this fear-based energy doing to humans who ingest it? I've often wondered if people who suffer from mood swings and depression would feel better if they eliminated this heavy energy from their diet.

I have a vegan friend whose daughter has cerebral palsy, and her ex-husband wanted the girl to eat meat. They asked Dr. Deepak Chopra about it, and he responded, "Meat is dead." End of story. Meat is dead, it is devoid of *prana*, life-force. Plants, on the other hand, have lots of prana.

In conjunction with your yoga pilot study, consider cutting out meat, fish, dairy, and eggs for thirty days. This will help you lose weight and feel energetically lighter and more connected to your soul and all beings. The former personal trainer in me would like to advise you to approach it Nike style and "Just Do It"… but I know this might not work for everyone. You can also take the approach of vegan authors— such as Kathy Freston, who says, "lean into it," or Alicia Silverstone, who says, "flirt with it."

It is hard to quit something when you are feeding it daily. Food addictions are like little Pac Mans in the body, waka-

wakaing around aimlessly, waiting to get their next fix. Here is an example: Junior Mints are my husband's favorite movie candy and, believe it or not, they are vegan. One time we were seeing a movie with teenage boy humor and my husband cracked up hysterically. At the same time, he sucked a whole Junior Mint down his wind pipe. I thought I was going to have to give him the Heimlich maneuver in the theater. He ran out into the lobby and I went chasing after him. Thank goodness, he coughed it up and was left standing there with a half box of uneaten candy. Like a good wife/mommy, I took them from him and went to throw them in the trash. He screamed, "NOOOOOOOOO!" just like a small child…and dove in front of the trash can to grab them out of my hand. I was mortified. He joyfully took them back into the theater like nothing had ever happened and finished the box. (You can tell my husband is the fun one in the family. Too bad he didn't write this book instead.)

This is an extreme example of what happens when you feed the sugar Pac Man within you. However, if you starve out cravings like sugar, meat, and dairy by not feeding them their food of choice, the addiction loses its power over you. Eventually it diminishes and then it's completely gone, like it was never even there in the first place. "I used to eat *what*?"

Chapter 12
Four Life-Changing Words: What Are You Eating?

Nothing's changed my life more. I feel better about myself as a person, being conscious and responsible for my actions, and I lost weight and my skin cleared up. I got bright eyes and I just became stronger and healthier and happier. I can't think of anything better in the world to be but be vegan.
—Alicia Silverstone

When I became vegetarian, I had never heard of "vegan." It turns out the word "vegan" was coined by Donald Watson of the UK in 1944. He defined it as "a way of living that seeks to exclude, as far as possible and practicable, all forms of, exploitation of, and cruelty to, animals for food, clothing, and any other purpose."

In 2002, a few years after turning vegetarian, I went to a Global Peace Alliance Conference at Marianne Williamson's church at the time, outside of Detroit. One of the guest speakers was Ohio Congressman Dennis Kucinich. He talked about his history of health problems and how his doctors couldn't come up with a diagnosis.

He then read John Robbins' best-selling book, *Diet for a New America,* which promoted a plant-based diet. John's dad, Irv Robbins, and his uncle were the founders of the billion-dollar Baskin Robbins ice cream empire. John grew up eating ice cream for breakfast and even had an ice-cream-cone-shaped swimming pool. His uncle died of a heart attack in his early fifties and his father developed high blood pressure and diabetes. According to John's son, Ocean Robbins, "You may know a little of our family story: My grandfather started Baskin-Robbins and groomed my dad to one day succeed him. My dad walked away from the family company and any access to his father's ice cream fortune. He followed his own 'rocky road' and devoted his life to advocating for health, compassion, and sustainability."

After Congressman Kucinich read *Diet for a New America*, he decided to adopt a plant-based diet, and his health started to improve dramatically. I was sitting in the audience, absorbing every word like a sponge. I had been suffering from acne, allergies, and asthma and was worried I was over-using my inhaler at night, which was giving me the shakes in my sleep. I thought, "Well, I'm already vegetarian. I'm almost there." I decided to eliminate eggs and dairy from my diet, and voilà! My acne, allergies, and asthma immediately dissipated.

I was upset that in all the years I had suffered from these ailments, neither my doctors nor dermatologists had ever asked me these four magic words, "WHAT ARE YOU EATING?" Instead they gave me prescriptions and sent me on my way.

The Power of a Plant-Based Diet for Health and Weight Loss

Some people think the plant-based, whole-foods diet is extreme. Half a million people a year will have their chests opened up and a vein taken from their leg and sewn onto their coronary artery. Some people would call that extreme.
—Dr. Caldwell Esselstyn, M.D., Author of *Prevent and Reverse Heart Disease*

Cardiologist Caldwell Esselstyn is featured in the documentary *Forks Over Knives,* which is an instant on

Netflix. This film examines the impact of a plant-based diet on controlling and even reversing diseases, such as heart disease, cancer, and diabetes. A plant-based diet is also extremely effective in helping people lower their cholesterol and blood pressure. In the film, doctors brilliantly take their patients to the grocery store and teach them how to shop for healthy food, instead of giving them more medications. These patients use the power of a plant-based diet, combined with exercise, to reduce their medications or to get off of them completely.

Dr. Neal Barnard, who thirty years ago founded the Physician's Committee for Responsible Medicine in Washington D.C., says, "The beef industry has contributed to more American deaths than all the wars of this century, all natural disasters, and all automobile accidents combined."

Forks Over Knives and the Physician's Committee both advocate a low fat, whole-foods, plant-based diet filled with vegetables, fruits, legumes (beans, peas and lentils), and complex carbohydrates. Yes, CARBS, JOY! We need carbs for energy and thyroid function. They are an important part of a balanced diet.

A plant-based diet is high in fiber, which can help eliminate wastes from the body, including excess weight, hormones, and residual medications. Meat is devoid of fiber. Plants also have protein, so you don't need to worry about not getting your protein fix. Beans, lentils, peas, nuts, nut butters, plant milks, tofu, brown rice, quinoa, and even vegetables are also a source of protein. In general, you don't need to eat an excessive amount of any type of protein, plant-based or animal-based. Too much protein slows down your digestion, is stressful on the kidneys and the liver, and can block your colon.

Animal products—even fish, lobster, shrimp, and crab—are filled with fat and cholesterol. Cholesterol comes from animal products, while plants have zero cholesterol. It's that simple. If you want to lower your cholesterol, don't eat foods with cholesterol. There are people who will naturally produce excessive cholesterol, due to hereditary factors. If this is the case for you, don't let your genetic predisposition get you down. Do your best to change to a plant-based diet and do your part to lower your cholesterol and improve your health.

One time I had my cholesterol checked and my doctor told me it was the lowest she'd ever seen—not dangerously low, just low. A cholesterol level of below 150 is considered ideal in the prevention of heart disease. I told her I was vegan and she said, "Nuts have cholesterol." This perplexed me, but because she was the doctor I listened to her. I went home and looked at the jar of peanut butter and it said, "0 cholesterol." Peanuts have fat, but no cholesterol. Only animal products have cholesterol. It's important to educate yourself on your nutritional choices and to choose doctors who have training in nutrition as well.

I met a woman who has Multiple Sclerosis who was part of a year-long study with Dr. John McDougall, a physician and leading proponent of vegan diets. She was in the control group that did not eat a vegan diet and was happy to keep eating animal products. She had no desire to change her diet at the time. At the end of the study, she still took her medicine like she always had. She was invited out to Dr. McDougall's center in California for a free 10-day in-patient trial. During the trial, she ate a low fat whole foods plant-based diet...and by the end of her visit, she was off her MS medicine completely. To this day, she doesn't need her medicine, unless she goes off her plant-based diet. Obviously, everyone's body chemistry is different, and some people may need medicine in conjunction with a plant-based diet, but it's sure worth the effort in changing your diet to see how food can impact your health. Dr. McDougall is known for saying, "It's the food." If you want to lose weight and improve your health, you must pay attention to your food.

In the '90s, I worked at the Pritikin Longevity Center in Santa Monica, which specialized in medical weight loss for people with health problems such as obesity, diabetes, high cholesterol, and high blood pressure. We had clients who weighed over 500 pounds and were in dire need of lifestyle changes. They were fed a low-fat, vegetarian diet and walked daily. I was amazed at how many people lost weight and were able to get off their cholesterol and blood pressure medications due to diet and exercise changes. It was powerful testimonial that food can be your medicine, if you give it a chance.

What Do Vegans Eat?

Could you look an animal in the eyes and say to it, "My appetite is more important than your suffering"?
—Moby

"What do you eat?" This is a common question asked by people who don't understand what it means to eat a vegan diet. There's a myth that vegans just eat iceberg lettuce salads and sprouts, which for my husband and me would be boring, sad, and leave us feeling like starving space cadets. Not to mention crabby, too. We eat lots of cooked food and a little raw food in addition to daily "treats" to satisfy the sweet cravings, like dates or black bean brownies. I have included a vegan recipe section in the back of the book to help give you ideas of delicious and satisfying recipes.

Basically, it's quite simple: To eat a vegan diet, you are just eliminating four things: meat, fish, dairy, and eggs. You can eat all the fruits, vegetables, grains, and legumes (beans, peas, lentils) you want. You can also eat small portions of nuts. They are high in fat and calories, so it's best to keep them to a minimum. Most of your favorite foods, recipes, and even baked goods can be "veganized." Meats can be replaced with veggie versions of bacon, sausage, hot dogs, and chicken, which are available in health food stores and some regular grocery stores. You can use veggie crumbles to replace ground hamburger. Most of these meat substitutes have gluten and soy in them. If you are sensitive to either of these foods, or you don't want your vegan meal to look or smell like meat, you could try adding some other forms of plant-based protein, such as beans, which are high in protein and fiber and low in fat and calories. Be sure and include a source of vitamin B12 in your diet, which can come from fortified cereals, soy milks or a supplement of five micrograms or more per day.

Breakfast
- Oatmeal or steel-cut oats, with plant milk, fresh fruit, maple syrup, and cinnamon
- Pancakes or waffles, with blueberries and maple syrup
- Cold grain cereal or granola with plant-based "milk" such as soy or almond
- Tofu scramble with toast and avocado spread. If you want "butter" on your toast, my favorite vegan butter is made by Earth Balance, which can also be used for baking.
- Whole grain toast with jam, apple butter, or your favorite nut butter such as peanut, almond, cashew, or sunflower. Look for nut butters in their pure form without added sugar. Many health food stores, such as Whole Foods, have the nut machines on display so you can grind your own fresh nut butter. Costco also sells no-sugar-added peanut butter,

which is delicious, once you adjust your taste buds to the lack of sugar.

Lunch
- Rice, tofu, and veggie bowls, with sesame dressing
- Spring rolls with peanut dipping sauce, veggie sushi
- Burritos with black beans, guacamole, lettuce, salsa (hold the cheese and sour cream)
- Veggie sandwiches on whole grain bread with your favorite veggies and lettuce, with hummus, mustard or vegan mayo (Veganaise and Just Mayo are good brands.)
- Big salads with colorful veggies, beans, nuts, fruits, avocado slices, and cubed baked tempeh or tofu. (You can buy packaged baked tofu with sauce on it, or you can bake your own.)
- Tofu eggless salad or chickpea salad on whole grain bread or a bed of kale, with crackers. These are easy meals to take to work with you for lunch.
- Bean chili and vegetables, with corn bread
- Carrot ginger soup
- Curry lentil, cauliflower, and spinach soup
- Baked potato with veggies and salsa
- Veggie burger, side salad, and baked sweet potato fries

Dinner
- Spinach lasagna, side salad, and garlic bread
- Sweet potato and black bean enchiladas
- Veggie fajitas with Spanish rice and black beans
- Quinoa and lentil tacos with kale, salsa, onions, and avocado slices
- Cauliflower Mac-'n-"Cheese," with a side of peas
- Stir-fry vegetables and tofu with Braggs Amino Acids or tamari sauce, both of which are gluten-free. Braggs Aminos has very low sodium. Soy sauce contains gluten.

- Falafel, hummus, and side salad
- Pasta with red sauce, veggies, and garlic bread
- Fettuccine with broccoli and vegan cheese Alfredo sauce
- Veggie pizzas, with extra sauce and favorite veggies; hold the cheese. (Most vegan cheese has a lot of oil and fat in it. I would omit it for weight loss. If you can't live without it, Daya is a popular brand of vegan shredded cheese, and Field Roast makes tasty vegan cheese slices. Check the ingredient label to make sure your vegan cheese is free of casein, the protein found in milk.)

Vegan cream sauces can be made in a blender, combining cashews, plant milk, and nutritional yeast. Nutritional yeast is full of B vitamins and looks like yellow flakes. It can be found in bulk at the health food store, or in a shaker form by Braggs. Make sure you don't buy Brewer's yeast, the kind used in baking, as it's much different.

Desserts
- Tofu chocolate mousse
- Oatmeal raisin cookies
- Chocolate chip cookies, using non-dairy chocolate chips
- Lemon cake, with lemon vegan cream cheese frosting
- Snickerdoodles
- Chocolate cake, with dark chocolate frosting
- Cookies 'n "cream" cupcakes

The list is endless.

Snacks
- Soy or coconut milk yogurt with fresh fruit
- Granola bars
- Banana blueberry smoothie with vanilla soy milk
- Apple slices, celery sticks, or rice cakes with peanut butter or almond butter

- Chopped veggies, crackers, rice cakes, and hummus
- Figs, dates, and raisins
- Small handfuls of almonds or cashews
- Dark chocolate squares
- Gluten-free crackers, such as Mary's Gone Crackers
- Pretzels
- Wheat Thins
- Rice Crackers and Corn Thins by Real Foods
- Air-popped popcorn with nutritional yeast

Eating Vegan in Social Gatherings

As I said in the beginning of the book, your food choices are something you control three times a day. *You* control it, not your family members, friends, co-workers, partners, children, or the media. Don't let them negatively influence or pressure you. No matter what other people are doing around you, practice strong will and speak up for your health, without making it a big deal. Just politely say "no, thank you" when needed and ask if there's a veggie option available. You can always bring your own food to a family barbeque, like a veggie burger and vegetarian baked beans. *Skinny Bitch in the Kitch* has a fantastic recipe for vegan potato salad. For dessert, you could bring a non-dairy ice cream made from soy, coconut, or rice milk. *So Delicious* is a yummy brand. For a holiday dinner, you could bring a few vegan side dishes and a dessert and make a meal out of them.

Another option is to plan ahead and eat a meal a few hours before a family dinner, work event, party, or wedding, so you're not starving, and then snack on any vegan options available. You can also call the host before the party and ask if there will be any vegan dishes being served and offer to bring one of your favorite vegan appetizers. If you're having a work party, bring a beautiful vegan dessert to share with your co-workers, like the decorative and delicious cupcakes from the cookbook, *Vegan Cupcakes Take Over the World* (now *that's* a book title!). I'm sure your co-workers will be pleasantly surprised how delicious they taste, even minus the animal products. Don't be afraid of being different from the crowd, and make your health a top priority. Your vegan choices may inspire those around you to make healthier choices as well. Lead by example, and don't take the meat jokes personally.

Eating Vegan in Restaurants

The easiest way to eat vegan out is to search in your area for vegan and vegetarian restaurants. There's also a web site called www.happycow.net that has a list of veggie- friendly restaurants internationally.

When dining out in a traditional restaurant, just ask for a vegan meal. I have found most restaurants will work with you, so feel free to ask for what you want. Millions of people have severe food allergies, and waiters are used to special requests. Just make sure you clarify that you don't want any dairy, eggs, meat, or fish. Not all servers understand what vegan means yet, but it is becoming more mainstream. I've had waiters say, "So that means you can eat fish?" Then I just politely explain what I can eat. You can also ask your server to omit the cheese, meat, and eggs from an existing entree or create your own meal according to the ingredients listed in various dishes. There might also be ingredients available in the kitchen that aren't listed on the menu. Be creative and have fun.

Look at the menu online before you go the restaurant and see what options are available to you. You can also call ahead and ask if the chef can prepare you a vegan meal. Ethnic restaurants—such as Chinese, Thai, Japanese, Mexican, Indian, Ethiopian, and Italian—are easier places to find vegan options than a steak house (obviously). If you have a set-back, don't beat yourself up. Your next meal is your point of power to begin again.

Hopefully you can see—and soon taste first-hand—that being vegan can be delicious and doesn't mean deprivation. There are numerous plant-based foods to be enjoyed and explored by your palate. It's going to take some effort and trial and error on your part to see what foods you like best, but you will learn a lot during the process.

Cooking for Yourself: Because You're Worth It

Learning to cook for yourself is life-changing. I didn't learn until my 40s and regret not learning sooner. My husband, Wade, has actually been my teacher. He taught himself how to cook after his divorce and gets better every year we've been married. I let him do the more complicated recipes and use him as a sounding board for cooking questions. I've learned that cooking is like anything else in life: it just takes practice. I started off slowly, but I can tell that with daily practice, I am getting better and faster. Don't give up if something doesn't turn out as expected. Check into vegan cooking classes at health food stores and hospitals, or vegan meet-up groups in your area. If you have any vegan friends, see if you can hang out in the kitchen and learn a few tricks from them. Host vegan potlucks in your community and build a group of like-minded new friends to support each other.

Do your grocery shopping on a different day from your cooking days, so you don't feel like food is consuming your life. Prep work like chopping vegetables, or making large pots of soup or a lasagna, can be done on the weekends to prepare for your work week. You can always freeze the leftovers and pull them out of your freezer as needed. Purchase a rice cooker for easy rice and quinoa cooking. They are inexpensive and simple to use: put two cups rice and three cups water into the cooker and turn it on. You will have perfect rice in just 20 minutes.

Pick basic recipes that are easy to follow, and keep practicing daily until you find your favorites dishes. *Oh She Glows* is my favorite vegan cookbook. Author Angela Liddon has outdone herself in creating crowd-pleasing vegan recipes your whole family will enjoy. Once you find your favorites— like her nacho dip, which is made from cashews, nutritional yeast, and carrots—you can introduce your friends and family to some fantastic new foods. My friend Star says, "That nacho dip changed my life." It's that crazy good!

My husband and I had a vegan wedding in 2008 in Santa Monica and invited our Midwest friends and relatives. They still rave about the food to this day (especially the wedding cake) which was all catered by Real Food Daily. When we went for our cake tasting, I was expecting to have five vegan flavors to pick from, but to my surprise there were close to 50 different flavors, including peanut butter and jelly. We chose "The Hawaiian," which was made with buckwheat flour and had grilled pineapple and coconut between the three layers and was topped with vegan buttercream icing. It was insane!

The creative chefs in the vegan baking world have it down. It's amazing what they can do without using eggs, milk, or butter. Look for a vegan bakery in your area. They are beginning to pop up everywhere, such as *Mud Pie Bakery* in Kansas City, Missouri, a city that is revered for its barbeque. The world is changing.

Got Zits? Get Glowing Skin from the Inside Out

I used to have terrible acne on my face, red, splotchy discoloration. And mucus—I was constantly blowing my nose. Then one day, this woman sits down next to me on a bus and says, "You're lactose intolerant." It all cleared up in three days. That changed my life. Doctors couldn't figure it out.
—Woody Harrelson

If you have acne, eliminate cow's milk and dairy products from your diet today. This is one of the best things you can do for your skin. When I was vegetarian, I ate an entire Chicago-style spinach-cheese dip at a restaurant, and the next day I had little pimples all over my face. My friend said, "The hormones from the dairy are coming out of your skin." I wanted to be sick.

If you are a woman, think about when you have a menstrual cycle acne flare-up. That is caused by the excess hormones in your body. The same thing happens when you consume dairy and meat products: You are consuming the naturally-occurring hormones from the animal, and, if the product is not organic, additional hormones that are induced by the farmers to fatten up the animals for slaughter. These excessive hormones detox out through your skin, causing acne.

Dairy milk is intended to grow a baby calf, not a person. Dairy milk is filled with hormones and sugar (lactose), and is considered "pregnant cow milk juice." It's good for growing a baby calf into a large cow within a year, not for your skin and body weight. Eliminating dairy products saved me from years of acne stress and embarrassment. The cycle of picking pimples and then spending hours trying to cover them up with make-up is no longer a ritual in my life.

My skin immediately cleared up when I went off dairy, and I bet your skin will, too. It doesn't take much dairy to kick up an acne episode in people who are prone to it, so do your best to stay COMPLETELY off dairy. Recurring acne can be detrimental to self-esteem for both teens and adults. I know it was a constant source of anxiety for me when I was young. I wish teenagers were taught the importance of nutrition for healthy skin in school to help them clear up acne and improve self-confidence. Eliminating sugar and caffeinated drinks will help as well.

Eating a plant-based diet, high in fiber, is also wonderful for getting your body cleansed from these excessive hormones and toxins. These foods act as colon-scrubbers, brushing the intestinal wall. Your skin will radiate health as a by-product of a clean diet and colon. Because your skin is your largest organ, it only makes sense that what you eat and drink can have a direct impact on your skin. Keeping drinking water as your main beverage.

There are many delicious forms of plant-based milks, such as soy, almond, cashew, coconut, hemp, oat, and rice. Almond, cashew, and soy milks are my favorite and can also be used in baking. Some plant milks are calcium-fortified. Keep in mind green vegetables, legumes, and tofu are also great sources of calcium. Try out several types and brands of plant milk and discover for yourself which ones satisfy your taste buds. Feel good knowing you are nourishing your body and helping your skin.

By choosing plant-based milks, you are helping to save dairy cows, who are repeatedly impregnated for the milk industry until they are physically spent and sent to slaughter. Their male babies are taken from them at birth for the veal industry and are bottle-fed by humans and not fed by their mothers. This causes the mothers to have deep grief and separation anxiety for their babies. They will often go looking for them, IF they have the freedom to roam. The calves who are often sold off to the veal industry are slaughtered at 18 to 20 weeks of age. This breaks my heart to even write these words. I had no idea of this cruelty before becoming vegan. I didn't understand the connection between the dairy and veal industries. I feel it is important for people to understand what is happening behind the scenes of their favorite dairy products, cheeses and yogurts, so they can be educated in their milk choices.

The terms "grass fed, humane, free-range and organic" don't mean cruelty-free. In the end, the animals are still being exploited and slaughtered.

My perspective of veganism was most affected by learning that the veal calf is a by-product of dairying, that in essence there is a slice of veal in every glass of what I had thought was innocuous white liquid—milk.
—Rynn Berry (Author of *Food for the Gods: Vegetarianism & the World's Religions*)

21-Day Vegan Cleanse
A bad habit can be quickly changed. A habit is the result of concentration of the mind. You have been thinking a certain way. To form a new and good habit, just concentrate in the opposite direction.
—Paramahansa Yogananda

Cleansing is a way to detoxify and rejuvenate the body. It releases toxins you have accumulated through food, environment, and product absorption. What you eat affects your physical health, your energy levels, the way you think, and your emotions. It's good from time to time to take a step back from your normal ways of eating and take inventory of the foods you are choosing to fuel your body temple. A cleanse can help you lose weight and also help with acne, eczema, allergies, asthma, arthritis, migraines, and digestion problems, all while boosting your immune system.

I host 21-day online vegan cleanses that are also gluten-free, caffeine-free, and alcohol-free. This is the way I live my life, and it has improved my health, skin, and spirit tremendously. I love helping people experience how easy and delicious it is to be vegan, without the need for stimulants. Many participants have stuck with this lifestyle after the cleanse ended because they feel so good. In just three weeks, people have lost up to10 pounds, simply from eating full vegan meals plus a few desserts…which even surprises me. I also encourage daily meditation, prayer, and exercise as a part of the cleanse.

This is not a limited calorie cleanse or a juice cleanse. This cleanse involves eating plant-based meals of your choice, so there's no deprivation or starvation. I don't tell people to count calories, either. Just eat a plant-based and gluten-free diet and it works, especially if you have weight to lose and are currently eating the standard American diet (SAD). Keep in mind that soda, chips, and Oreos are vegan, so you do have to make effort not to be a junk food vegan!

In addition to losing weight on the cleanse, participants tell me they feel more clear-headed and are sleeping better due to the caffeine being out of their system. Some people discover they are gluten-sensitive and didn't realize it until they eliminated gluten from their diet. One participant used to have abdominal pain and didn't know why. When she did the cleanse it went away, but when she reintroduced a piece of gluten bread, the pain came back. I also had a student whose severe eczema cleared up when she switched to a vegan and gluten-free diet and underwent a series of colonics.

Being gluten-free means you can still eat all your favorite carb foods such as bread, pasta, cereal, and crackers. Just switch them to gluten-free products and don't go crazy eating them. I lost five pounds when I went gluten-free, and I wasn't trying to lose weight. I don't have Celiac disease, but I do feel better when I don't eat gluten products. When I do eat them, it makes my nose stuffy and my chest congested. Like many people, I ate gluten my whole life and never had a problem until the last six years. Now I have switched all my wheat products to rice products, and I feel much better. The gluten-free market has become a billion dollar industry because so many people have become gluten sensitive.

I would love you to do my three-week cleanse to see if you notice a difference in your health, weight, moods, sleep, and thinking. After 21 days, if you don't think you are sensitive to gluten and want it back in your diet, slowly reintroduce it first, before anything else like caffeine or dairy, and see what happens. If you're fine with the reintroduction of gluten, focus on eating whole grain wheat products to get the benefit of the fiber, such as Ezekiel bread products.

In addition, focus on eating a variety of beans and lots of colorful fruits and vegetables with your meals. Strive to eat all the colors of the rainbow on a daily basis. I know this sounds like a kindergarten teacher, but when my step-daughter brought home a placemat that said, "Eat the colors of the rainbow," I realized my favorite foods were the color of the palm of my hand, like cereals, crackers, and rice. They were definitely not on the rainbow color chart. I now make an effort to incorporate as many colors as possible into my diet, which allows me to experience different flavorful and nutrient rich foods.

Chapter 13
Letting Go of the Love Affair with Caffeine

As I began to tune into my body and provide it with what it really wanted—fresh, whole, real, unprocessed foods; sleep, relaxation and the time to enjoy the life I had created for myself and my family—I was able to break up with coffee and make up with my health.
—Dr. Mark Hyman, M.D.

I drank coffee for 20 years, so I understand this addiction on a deep level. I don't win a lot of friends when I ask people to quit caffeine because it is socially encouraged, accepted, and HUGELY addictive. Caffeine can affect the quality of your skin, causing acne, dehydration, and dark circles under the eyes. It also causes imbalances in your blood sugar, which can cause cravings for sugary and fattening foods. Caffeine also increases the stress hormone cortisol in the body, which can cause you to overeat, and leads to weight gain over time.

Caffeine also increases blood pressure and heart rate, especially for those who aren't habitual coffee drinkers. It is acidic and can cause inflammation in the body, which can be harmful, especially if you have a health condition, joint problems, or are trying to heal an injury. Caffeine is a powerful drug; its side effects shouldn't be taken lightly.

Caffeine can affect your consciousness and altar your personality, causing mood swings, irritability, and impatience. Have you ever found yourself agitated soon after your morning coffee? If you find yourself having outbursts at a family member, your pet, a co-worker, or a stranger on the road, just know the caffeine could be altering your personality.

In my early years of teaching yoga, I would drink coffee before class and abrupt things would fly out my mouth, as if I were a crack addict. I would shake my head and think to myself, "Who is this person saying these things?" I now realize it was because my mind was filled with caffeine—drugs, basically. Remember those commercials, "This is your brain on drugs"? That is the way I felt, altered and not my best Self.

Later, in my 40s, when coffee and I were no longer "besties," I witnessed some of my coffee-drinking students having similar problems with moodiness. I found it hard to teach students who were caffeinated because I felt like there was a barrier between us. Who is the Self, when it is caffeinated?

I know quitting coffee may appear impossible, but once you get over the first few days and the possibility of a headache, you are home free. It's actually liberating not being controlled by a substance of any sort, knowing you don't need it to function throughout your day. If you are tired, take a quick, 10-minute nap to rejuvenate, go on a walk, or march in place to wake up. *You* are in control, not the addiction. Meditation will teach you that your mind aligned with Divine mind is more powerful than any drug or addiction. God has healed millions of people from addiction and He can do the same for you. Your meditation practice will also be deeper because you won't have the caffeine barrier between you and God. It's hard to be still and surrender when you're amped on caffeine.

When I look back on my relationship with coffee, I realize I was more addicted to the ritual of having something warm, sweet, and nurturing in my mug, than to the actual caffeine pulsing through my veins at night. According to Dr. Neal Barnard, "As much as one-quarter of the caffeine in your morning coffee is still circulating in your blood stream twelve hours later." If you suffer from insomnia, eliminate ALL caffeine—including chocolate—from your diet, and see if it helps you sleep. Meditate before bed as well.

There are delicious caffeine-free teas that can replace your morning ritual so you can still have something warm and fun in your mug. My favorite is Firelight Chai, by Zhena's Gypsy Tea. I drink it with a little steamed vanilla soy and cinnamon, and it's heaven in my cup. You can find it in the health food store or order it online. Numi Tea also makes a wonderful caffeine-free chai. There are also several brands of Rooibos teas, which you can doctor the same way. Celestial Tea makes several flavors of fruit teas such as lemon, peppermint, or mandarin orange, which are great alone. You can also drink warm lemon water with a splash of Bragg's Apple Cider Vinegar, which is helpful to balance out the pH in the body and cleanse the liver.

If you want a more coffee-tasting option, Teeccino is a popular herbal coffee alternative made from carob, barley, chicory, and ramen seeds. They have 18 flavors to choose from, including French Roast. They have it in tea bags or granule form, so you can scoop it into your coffee maker. My clients like the granule form better. You can use it to help wean yourself off caffeine, drinking it either alone or combining it with coffee.

There is an article on the Teeccino website about the negative impact caffeine has on weight loss, which is documented by medical research: www.teeccino.com/building_optimal_health/129/Caffeine-and-Weight-Loss.html

Drink caffeine-free tea or Teeccino in the morning and drink water the rest of your day. If you have a soda or diet soda addiction, try drinking one or two La Croix flavored waters a day instead. Purified water is better for your health and weight loss than carbonated water, so make it your number one beverage.

Chapter 14
Alcohol: You Won't Miss It

I'm very serious about no alcohol, no drugs. Life is too beautiful.
—Jim Carrey

My sweet dad, whom I loved dearly, was a Type II diabetic, which means his diabetes was induced by his food and drink choices. He was addicted to food, mostly animal products, and refused to change his diet and quit drinking alcohol. Alcohol and diabetes don't mix well together. He even had a polite wake-up call from the heavens that caused him to have both carotid arteries cleaned out due to a minor stroke. Still he wouldn't change. He ended up having a heart attack and dying in his sleep when he was 67 years old. He just didn't wake up on Easter morning. He missed out on a lot of beautiful memories in his future, including his 50th wedding anniversary, watching his grandkids grow up, and walking me down the aisle.

Even if my father had never had a drop of alcohol, I still wouldn't be a fan of it. I drank enough in my 20s to realize nothing good ever came from it. Plus, yoga and a hangover don't mix well. I learned this the hard way after having margaritas on my 30th birthday and showing up the next morning for my 7 a.m. yoga practice. My teacher said bluntly, "Alcohol is poison." She was right.

Alcohol, like caffeine, is a powerful drug and is toxic to your liver and body temple. I now think of it as drinking gasoline or fingernail polish remover. It is also filled with sugar and unnecessary calories. I had a yoga student show up to class looking leaner than I'd ever seen her in the past. She told me she had stopped drinking her two glasses of red wine a night, which equaled around 500 calories.

Alcohol also impairs your consciousness—which is, sadly, why many people drink: to escape their reality. Alcohol, like food, can be an escape mechanism when life throws people a curve ball and they want to numb their feelings. Instead of sitting with their emotions and working through them, alone or with another person, they go running to the refrigerator or alcohol to avoid the situation and any feelings of inadequacies, fear, stress, and anxiety.

When it comes to clear communication with friends, family members, and partners, make sure you aren't clouded by alcohol, so they have the pleasure of speaking to the *real* you, not the altered version of you. This will help your conversations to be more authentic and beneficial to all involved. Emotions can get heated when alcohol is involved. It's better to not to put fuel on the fire by drinking it.

Alcohol also acts as a barrier between your soul and God. If you are serious about deepening your spiritual connection and evolving your consciousness, it's a good idea to let go of alcohol permanently. Instead of self-medicating, sit in meditation and pray for strength, guidance, and clarity. Give God all your stressful feelings and ask for them to be healed. Take slow, deep breaths to quiet your mind, calm your nervous system, and connect with your soul.

You can also go for a walk outside and talk through your issues with God. I know this takes a lot of will power, but it sure beats hurting your body temple with excessive food, alcohol, and caffeine when you're already feeling vulnerable. Human beings can be masochistic in their need to self-destruct when they are stressed or want to relax. These are the times when we should be loving and nurture ourselves instead. Take a bath, call a trusted friend, spend time with your pet, or write in your journal. Keep reminding yourself that things always work out in time, that they always have and always will. What can seem catastrophic in the moment can, many times, have a silver lining in the end. Trust that God has the perfect plan for your life.

Chapter 15
Sadhana: Daily Spiritual Practice

Sadhana is self-enrichment. It is not something which is done to please somebody or to gain something. Sadhana is a personal process in which you bring out your best.
—Yogi Bhajan

In yoga, the term *sadhana* means spiritual practice, a daily routine of disciplines to help advance you on your personal and spiritual path. It can be done alone and/or with a group. It helps you stay true to yourself first, before you go about life's daily duties. Most spiritual disciplines begin early in the morning, so the first step is to get a good night's sleep. If you have a family to take care of in the morning, get up an hour earlier than your children for your alone time. You have to put yourself first. No one else will do it for you. The more you give to yourself, the more you will have to give to those around you.

In this program, your daily spiritual practice consists of the following:

- First thing in the morning, pray and meditate 5-20 minutes.
- Practice yoga 30+ minutes, depending on time constraints.

- Say your affirmations while you're getting ready for your day, while looking at yourself in the mirror. Examples: "I deeply and completely love and accept myself." "I am worthy and deserving of my heart's desires."
- Eat a healthy vegan breakfast, with caffeine-free tea or warm lemon water.
- Drink water throughout your day, especially before a meal and any time you have an empty stomach, but not while you eat.
- Bring a vegan lunch to work.
- During your lunch break, or later in the afternoon, take a 30-minute walk in nature to clear your mind and lift your vibration.
- In the evening, cook yourself a vegan dinner, play some music, light candles, and nurture your body temple with delicious plant-based foods.
- Journal before bed and write down anything that triggered you on an emotional level. How was your relationship with yourself and food on this day?
- Meditate again before bed, and pray, giving thanks for the day's events and the gift of being alive.

New habits take time and perseverance. Whether you start with the whole sadhana practice or just part of it, make your spiritual connection a top priority. Talk to God throughout your day, asking to be guided and blessed, and ask whom can you serve. Having this strong foundation will give you more discipline and help you control your emotions and cravings. Keep touching base with yourself to see how you are feeling and what beliefs are influencing your life. Allow your yoga practice to help you heal your relationship with yourself. In turn, this will help you heal your relationship with your body and food.

You're On Your Way to Permanent Weight Loss!

It is traditional to end a yoga class with the word *Namasté*, which simply translates to: "The Divine in me honors the Divine in you."

So I now say to you—Namasté. I see in you all that is good and light. Whether you believe it or not, it is there. And the more you see it, too, the happier you will be and the faster you will lose weight. I know this is going to be a life-changing journey for you. I applaud you for your efforts in being willing to change. Keep loving yourself lean!

Let's chat to see how I can support you

I want to help you feel empowered in your ability to manage your weight for life.

Contact me for a FREE discovery session to discuss your weight loss goals. www.kathleenkastner.com/; kathleen@kathleenkastner.com

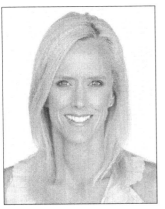

Kathleen Kastner has a master's degree in exercise physiology and is a wellness coach and yoga instructor. She is also a certified Food for Life plant-based instructor with the Physician's Committee for Responsible Medicine. Her celebrity clients have included Deepak Chopra, Molly Sims and Emily Deschanel. She lives in Encinitas, California.

Appendix 1
Resources

Yoga

www.kathleenkastner.com
Ashtanga videos, workshops and teacher trainings

www.ashtangayogacenter.com
Ashtanga workshops, teacher trainings, retreats and classes
with Tim Miller

www.omkar108.com
Ashtanga classes and retreats with Jorgen Christiansson

www.ashtanga.net
Ashtanga workshops, DVDs and Practice Manual by David
Swenson

www.yogavibes.com (Free two-week trial)
Ashtanga Full Primary Series by Wade Mortenson
Vinyasa videos by Kathleen Kastner and Wade Mortenson

Vegan Cookbooks and Blogs

Crazy, Sexy, Kitchen, by Kris Carr: www.kriscarr.com
The Beauty Detox Diet, by Kimberly Snyder:
www.kimberlysnyder.com
Oh She Glows, by Angela Liddon: www.ohsheglows.com
Bitchin Dietician, www.bitchindietician.com, by Jennifer K. Riley
R.D., L.D.
Positively Vegan, www.positivelyvegan.blogspot.com, by Kim Miles

Skinny Bitch in the Kitch, by Rory Freedman and Kim Barnouin, www.skinnybitch.net/
The Engine 2 Diet, by Rip Esselstyn: www.engine2diet.com
Forks Over Knives: www.forksoverknives.com
The China Study Cookbook, by Leanne Campbell, Ph.D.
Vegan Cupcakes Take Over the World, by Isa Chanda Moskowitz and Terry Hope Romero
The Joy of Vegan Baking, by Colleen Patrick Goodreau

Meditation

A Path with Heart, by Jack Kornfield
How To Meditate: A Practical Guide to Making Friends with Your Mind, by Pema Chödrön
Meditations for Weight Loss, by Marianne Williamson (Audible)
Insight Timer - Meditation application

Life-Changing Films

Forks Over Knives: A documentary promoting the benefits of eating a plant-based diet: Netflix or www.forksoverknives.com

Cowspiracy: The effects of animal agriculture on the environment: Netflix or www.cowspiracy.com

Earthlings: A documentary about the suffering of animals for food: fashion, pets, entertainment, and medical research. Narrated by Joaquin Phoenix. Available to watch at: www.earthlings.com

Ashtanga NY: A documentary of Pattabhi Jois' visit to New York City during 9-11. Available at: firstrunfeatures.com/cgi-bin/sc/productsearch.cgi?storeid=*100b93576b06b5905e02

Crazy Sexy Cancer: Kris Carr's documentary on living with cancer and treating it with a plant-based diet: Netflix or www.kriscarr.com

Appendix 2
Recipes

Steel Cut Oats (2 servings—cut in half for one person)
Ingredients:
3 cups water
1 cup steel cut oats
Handful of blueberries
Small handful of chopped pecan or walnuts
Splash of almond milk or other plant milk
1 Tbsp. maple syrup or brown sugar
Cinnamon to top

Directions:
Combine water and oats in pot and bring to a boil. Cover and simmer on low for 30 minutes. Add fruit and nut toppings, maple syrup, almond milk, cinnamon. Devour and enjoy.

Oats by nature are gluten-free, but they can become cross-contaminated with other grains during processing. If you need a guaranteed gluten-free oat, Bob's Red Mill makes them.

Raw Oats (1 serving)
Ingredients:
½ bowl raw oats, regular or gluten-free
Plant milk to cover oats
Raisins or favorite fruit
1-2 Tbsp. maple syrup

Directions:

Pour oats and favorite plant milk in bowl. Top with raisins, blueberries, or other fruits and maple syrup.

All-The-Rage Baked Oatmeal (8 servings—can be reheated for later)
Prep Time: 5 minutes

Ingredients:
3 Tbsp. flaxseed meal (finely ground flax seeds)
1/4 cup warm filtered water
2 cups quick-cooking oats
1 cup rolled oats
1/2 cup packed brown sugar (optional)
2 tsp. baking powder
1/2 tsp. cinnamon
3/4 tsp. salt
1/4 tsp. ground ginger
1 cup unsweetened almond milk or soy milk
2 Tbsp. Earth Balance margarine, melted
1/2 cup fresh blueberries (preferably organic)
6 chopped fresh strawberries (preferably organic)

Directions:
Preheat the oven to 350 F. Lightly oil an 8" square or round baking pan. In a small bowl, combine the flax meal with the warm water until the mixture forms a gel. Set aside 5 minutes.

In a medium-sized bowl, combine the quick-cooking oats, rolled oats, brown sugar, baking powder, cinnamon, salt, and ginger. Set aside. In another small mixing bowl, whisk together the almond milk and melted margarine. Add this to the dry ingredients, followed by the flax mixture. Stir until just combined. Fold in the blueberries and strawberries until evenly distributed.

Spread the mixture in the prepared pan and bake for 35-40 minutes, or until a toothpick inserted in the center emerges clean. Cut into 8 squares and serve warm with almond milk or soy milk.

Recipe reprinted with permission from:
bitchindietitian.com/2012/03/01/baked-oatmeal-everyones-doing-it/

Buckwheat Flour Pancakes
Serves 2-3 people (8 medium-sized pancakes)
Buckwheat flour is gluten-free if you buy it in bulk. However, most premade buckwheat pancake mixes are in a box contain wheat, so read the label.

Ingredients:
1 1/4 cup buckwheat flour (For best results use buckwheat flour, not other flours.)
2 tsp. baking powder
1 tsp. cinnamon
1 1/4 cup almond or soy milk
1 tsp. vanilla extract
1 Tbsp. vegetable oil
2 Tbsp. Maple syrup

Directions:
Combine dry ingredients. Add the remaining ingredients and whisk well, but do not over-mix. Let stand for a minute.

Pour batter into 4 cakes until browned on each side. Then repeat with 4 more cakes. If you don't have a nonstick pan, you can use extra coconut oil in the pan. Serve with maple syrup and blueberries.

Banana Peanut Butter Smoothie (1 serving)
(For nut allergies, substitute blueberries, strawberries, or peaches)

Ingredients:
1 cup almond or soy milk
1 frozen or non-frozen banana (Peel and chop bananas and store in freezer bag to keep on hand.)
1 Tbsp. natural peanut butter
1 stalk kale (optional)

Directions:
Blend all ingredients for 30-60 seconds. Drink immediately.

Nature's Path Products:
Mesa Sunrise gluten-free cereal
Flax Plus or Pumpkin Flax Granola
Wildberry or Pumpkin Waffles: frozen and gluten-free (add a little peanut butter and syrup).

LUNCH & DINNER

Super Simple Oil-Free Kung Pao
(3 servings)
Set 1 cup dry brown rice or quinoa to cook while you make the sauce and chop the vegetables. (Read the directions on the package of rice or use a rice cooker.)

Sauce:

1 Tbsp. arrowroot

1/2 cup water

1 Tbsp. fresh grated ginger

1 Tbsp. fresh minced garlic

1/4 cup toasted sesame tahini

3 Tbsp. tamari, or to taste (use the low sodium kind if you can get it)

3 T maple syrup

1 T umeboshi plum paste

1 T Sriracha sauce

1 T white vinegar

Place the arrowroot in a medium sized bowl. Slowly whisk in the water until well-blended, with no lumps. Add the remaining ingredients and whisk until blended. Set aside.

Veggies:

1/2 yellow onion, chopped

2 carrots, chopped

1/2 cup raw cashews or peanuts, chopped

1/2 tsp. red pepper flakes

2 cups cooked rice or quinoa

1 bunch broccoli, cut into small florets

Sauté onion in a little water, over medium-high heat, for 2-3 minutes.

Add the carrots, nuts, pepper flakes, and rice, and cook for 2-3 minutes more, adding a little more water if the rice sticks.

Add the broccoli and cook for 1-2 minutes, just until it turns bright green.

Pour the sauce over the veggies, but do not stir in yet.

Quickly cover the pan, turn off the heat, and leave it to steam for 5-10 minutes. Stir before serving.

Top with more nuts, hot sauce, or red pepper flakes for extra heat.

Recipe reprinted with permission from:
positivelyvegan.blogspot.com/2013/03/super-simple-oil-free-kung-pao.html

Walnut Burgers (3 or 4 servings)
Ingredients:
1 cup walnuts, toasted and chopped
1/2 cup cooked quinoa
1/2 cup onion, finely chopped
1/2 cup bread crumbs
1 Tbsp. dry basil
1/4 tsp. powdered sage
1/4 tsp. powdered thyme
1/2 tsp. salt
1/4 tsp. pepper
1 tsp. vegan Worcestershire
3 Tbsp. tomato paste
3 Tbsp. flaxseed meal mixed with 3 Tbsp. water

Directions:
Mix all ingredients in a large bowl with your hands. Shape into 3 or 4 patties. Fry in a non-stick pan over medium heat, until browned on both sides.

Recipe reprinted with permission from:
positivelyvegan.blogspot.com/search?q=walnut+burger

Accidental Lentil Stew (8 hearty servings, about 1 cup each)
Ingredients:
4 cups filtered water
1 16-ounce (1 lb.) bag dried red split lentils
8 oz. organic frozen chopped spinach (or other dark leafy green; use half of a 16 oz. bag)
2 garlic cloves, minced (I used 2 Dorot frozen garlic cubes)
1/2 tsp. ground ginger
1 tsp. curry powder
1 tsp. sea salt (or more to taste)

Directions:
Place all ingredients in a medium-size soup pot and simmer for 15 minutes. Serve with bread, multigrain crackers, or nothing at all.
Recipe reprinted with permission from:
bitchindietitian.com/2012/11/17/accidental-lentil-stew/

Veggie Pizza
Ingredients:
Pizza crust, regular or gluten-free. (Most health food stores and some pizza restaurants will sell ready made gluten-free crusts. Mama Mary's pizza crusts are vegan and some are gluten-free.)
Marinara sauce
Broccoli
Red, yellow, or orange peppers
Purple onion
Additional favorite veggies

Directions:
Place sauce and veggies on crust and bake according to directions.

Optional vegan parmesan topping: 1 cup cashews, 1-2 Tbsp. nutritional yeast, and ½ tsp. salt; process all ingredients in high powered blender.

Quick and Easy Bean Burritos and Tostados - Simple and Fast

Ingredients:
Corn tortillas or corn tostado shells
Refried vegetarian black or pinto beans
Chopped white onions, tomato, lettuce/kale,
Avocado slices
Salsa

Directions:
Heat tortillas or bake tostado shells according to directions. Fill with warm beans and top with veggies, avocado, and salsa

SIDE DISHES

Easy Guacamole

Ingredients:
3-5 ripe avocados
1/2 cup chopped Vidalia or other sweet onion
1 clove of garlic, pressed or minced
1 Tbsp. of lemon juice
1/2 tsp. sea salt
1 Roma tomato, chopped (optional)

Directions:
Mash avocados in a mixing bowl with the back of a spoon or fork. Stir in the rest of the ingredients. Serve with chips and salsa or add as a topping to burritos, tostados, or tacos. Cover

leftovers with cellophane pressed down against the guacamole, with no air gap. Eat leftovers within 1-2 days.

Baked Cinnamon Sweet Potato Fries (3 servings)
Ingredients:
2 large sweet potatoes or 3 medium ones
2 Tbsp. olive oil
Generous amount of cinnamon
Dash of black pepper
Dried thyme
Ketchup and hot sauce (optional)

Directions:
Preheat oven to 425 degrees. Peel sweet potatoes; be sure to remove any dark spots.

Cut sweet potatoes into strips about 2-3 times the thickness of a traditional French fry and put them in the largest mixing bowl you have. Pour in enough olive oil to coat the entire fry surface (start with a little olive oil, and add more as needed). Then sprinkle on the cinnamon (be generous) and a few dashes of black pepper.

Now…time to get messy. Use your hands to toss the fries with the oil and spices. After turning things over a few times, add more cinnamon, pepper, and thyme. When you can see that all the cinnamon is wet with a complete coating of oil over the fried, spread the fries evenly on a cookie sheets and put them in the oven for 30-45 minutes, depending on how thickly you sliced them. To test for doneness, put a fork in one of the fat ones to make sure it is soft all the way through.

Enjoy with a little ketchup and maybe some hot sauce.

Slow Baked Yams or Sweet Potatoes (2 servings)
Ingredients:
2 yams or sweet potatoes

Directions:
Preheat oven to 350 degrees. Then cut the sweet potatoes into halves, wrap with foil, and bake for 60 minutes. They will slow-bake in their own sugar. Great for a snack or side dish.

Oven Roasted Brussels Sprouts (4 servings)
Ingredients:
1 lb. Brussels sprouts, rinsed and cut into halves
Olive oil
Sesame seeds
Garlic salt

Directions:
Preheat oven to 400 degrees. Place halves of Brussels sprouts in bowl and lightly drizzle with olive oil. Sprinkle with garlic salt and sesame seeds; toss with hands to coat sprouts. Place in a single layer on cookie sheet. To avoid sticking, you can cover the cookie sheet with tinfoil or parchment, but it will work fine either way. Bake for 25 minutes.

Clean Bean Casserole (Serves 8)

Creamy Mushroom Gravy:
1 cup raw cashews, submerged in water and soaked overnight (or at least 4 hours)
1 Tbsp. olive oil
20 oz. sliced white mushrooms
2 cloves garlic, minced
1 vegetable bouillon cube

"Fried" Onions:
1 large onion, sliced into crescents
¼ cup almond meal
1 Tbsp. cornstarch
½ tsp. black pepper
½ tsp. salt
2 Tbsp. olive oil

Green Beans:
2 lbs. green beans, ends removed

Directions:
Preheat oven to 350°

Mushroom gravy: Place soaked cashews into a blender of food processor along with the water they soaked in. Blend to make a "cream." Set aside. Heat oil in sauté pan and sauté mushrooms and garlic until cooked through. Add cashew "cream" and bouillon cube and continue to cook over medium heat until bouillon cube dissolves. Set aside.

Onions: In a medium-sized bowl, combine almond meal, cornstarch, black pepper, and salt. Stir in the sliced onions until well-coated. In a sauté pan, heat olive oil and "fry" coated onions. Set aside.

Green beans: Place green beans into a 13 X 9-inch baking dish (pre-steam them for softer beans). Pour creamy mushroom mixture over top and stir to coat green beans. Top with onions and bake, uncovered, for 30 minutes.

Recipe reprinted with permission from:
bitchindietitian.com/2014/11/21/clean-bean-casserole/

DESSERTS

Oatmeal & Date Bites
Ingredients:
¾ cup pitted dates
1 cup raisins
2 cup oats (gluten-free if needed)
1 tsp. ginger
1 tsp. allspice
2 Tbsp. honey or agave nectar

Directions:
Put dates into food processor and pulse with 1-2 tsp. water.
Then add raisins and puree. Add oats and spices; process until
it turns thick and doughy. Roll into balls and serve.

Easy Chocolate Mousse (4 Servings)
Ingredients:
1 package silken tofu
1 ripe banana
2 Tbsp. unsweetened cocoa powder (most stores carry
Hershey's)
1 tsp. vanilla
2 Tbsp. maple syrup
Raspberries or strawberries (optional)

Directions:
Blend all ingredients in a blender and refrigerate. Top with a
raspberry or strawberry.

Lokah Samastah Sukhino Bhavantu

May all beings everywhere be happy and free, and may the thoughts, words, and actions of my own life contribute in some way to that happiness and to that freedom for all.

Thank you for caring!

33325576R00069

Made in the USA
San Bernardino, CA
29 April 2016